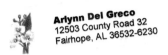
Arlynn Del Greco
12503 County Road 32
Fairhope, AL 36532-6230

Alive Polarity:
Healing Yourself and Your Family

ALIVE POLARITY:
Healing Yourself and Your Family

by

Jefferson Campbell
and the Alive Polarity Staff

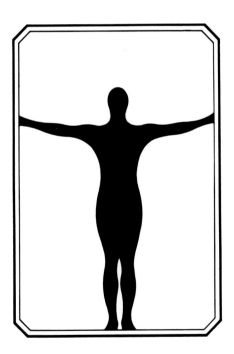

Alive Polarity Publications
Murrieta Hot Springs, Murrieta, California

Alive Polarity Publications
Murrieta Hot Springs
Murrieta, CA 92362

This work is the first volume in a series sponsored
by the Alive Fellowship and published by Alive
Polarity Publications.

Credits:
Edited by Judith Handelsman
Illustrated by Mark Allison
Co-ordinated by Ted Gruberman

ISBN: 0-941732-00-2 (hardcover);
ISBN: 0-941732-01-0 (softcover).

Library of Congress Catalog Number: 81-70027

Printed in the United States of America
First Printing, June 1982, 5,000 copies
Second Printing, May 1984, 5,000 copies
Third Printing, September 1985, 5,000 copies

With His grace, I dedicate this book
to my mother and father, Sharon, Liza,
Peter, and the Alive Fellowship.

CONTENTS

Most terms are defined extensively in the text. Words that are commonly used in everyday language such as "form" and "space" have very specific, and often different, meanings in Alive Polarity terminology. Use the Glossary as an aid when reading the chapters and enjoy it as a teaching tool by itself.

Charts

Art Work

Alive Polarity:
Healing Yourself and Your Family

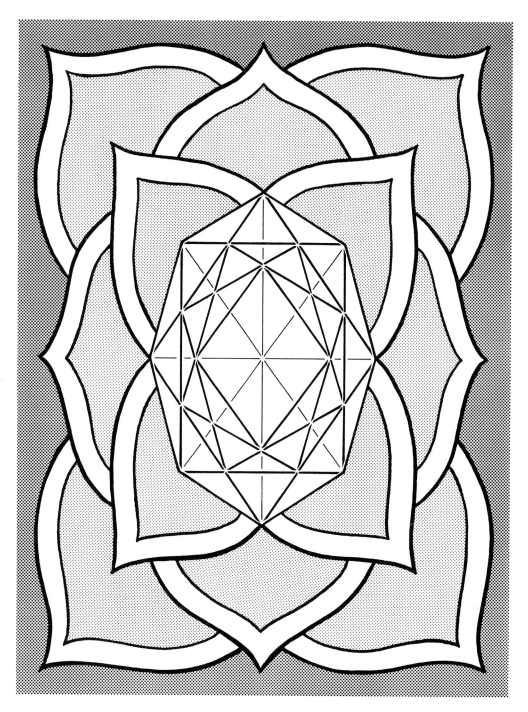

The diamond soul, or the jewel in the
lotus, symbol of awakened consciousness and balance.

I

Man and Woman:
The Essence of Alive Polarity

In this book I want to give an understanding of life which I call Alive Polarity. This understanding is the basis of all my work and I believe it is the key to the psychology and medicine of the Aquarian Age just as it was the key to these arts in the ancient past.

My goal is to transmit the essence of Alive Polarity in a practical way that can help us live in this world of duality and limitation while also realizing our soul. The core of this work is understanding the basic polarity and limitation of human life on this earth: what it means to be a man or a woman and how that fact relates to the soul inside us.

The male or female bodies we have are space suits that our souls have taken on in order to be able to live in this world and experience its duality and limitation. What gives these bodies life is the energy of the soul. Understanding how this soul energy manifests is the subject of this book.

The key to Alive Polarity is to understand and accept that we each have a man and a woman operating within us. We have a masculine side and a feminine side doing an elaborate dance, jockeying for the dominant position of the moment. Alive Polarity teaches us how these masculine and feminine energies function at their fullest potential, according to their specific natures, and how we can best utilize these energies in our lives.

For me, the two words "Alive Polarity" say it all. They sum up our whole situation. "Alive" describes the soul. The soul is the part of ourselves that is conscious of a reality beyond ourselves, conscious of the force that is pulling us out of this world and into the unknown out of which we have come. We can call this force God, the Lord, or whatever we choose. It is life, the essential energy we share with everything that breathes: trees, plants, insects, birds, animals, and all human beings on this planet.

"Polarity" describes the part of ourselves that exists in duality in the physical world. It is the part of ourselves that reacts to the world and is involved in the constant push-pull of cause and effect that keeps us in the world. Our duality begins with the reaction which produces us when the male sperm of our father enters the female egg of our mother. From that moment of conception our male and female parts begin to take form. After birth, from the time of our first thought, the domino theory takes over. One thought leads to another, each action leads to a reaction, reaction piles on top of reaction, and soon we become crystallized into a man-woman or a woman-man, depending on the body we choose.

In the human body we live in a world of limitation and pain. If we learn to work with the pain and accept what it is giving us, then we will be able to go beyond the limitations. Only then will we see the world as a learning place. It is actually a school where we may learn about ourselves and become more conscious of our soul, our life, and our true identity.

The more we resist our limitations, the more reaction we create in the form of emotions like hate, anger, fear, and attachment to people and things. These reactions perpetuate our pain and unconsciousness because we become lost in the emotions and lose contact with the clear light of our soul quality. Many people today are struggling with the situation of being caught in the web of their emotions and yet seeking the freedom of greater consciousness, greater realization of their soul quality. That soul quality is the consciousness and life that resides inside us. It is the part of ourselves we need to nurture.

Paradoxically, freedom comes from accepting the limitations of life in this human form, accepting the events and reactions in our lives and accepting our emotions. As we finally begin to accept our emotions and our limitations, we begin to concentrate and focus. Gradually our understanding increases, and with it, our humility. We truly experience what is called life. We know what it means to feel alive.

Looking at ourselves is the best way I know to understand our own limitations. At the time of conception, we either become more like our mothers and take on a female body, or we become more like our fathers and take on a male body. At that time we take on our sexual identity, our primary energy, and become a man or a woman, even though we always have both maleness and femaleness inside us.

It is ironic that in the midst of a sexual revolution people have such difficulty acknowledging their sexual identity. We need to accept that we all have a dominant sexual energy and that it is determined by our bodily form. Primarily, we are either a man or a woman and we have the other secondarily. Both are living together within us.

The *I-Ching* describes the male and female energies and their interrelationship in life so that we may understand the difference in their essential natures. Within the symbol of the *Tao*, it is clear that the spiralling masculine (*yang*) and feminine (*yin*) energies fit together perfectly in one circular form. They are not opposites, nor are they equal. Rather, they are complementary. Within the form of one is the seed of the other. That's what the dot signifies inside each half. Within their duality is harmony and completion.

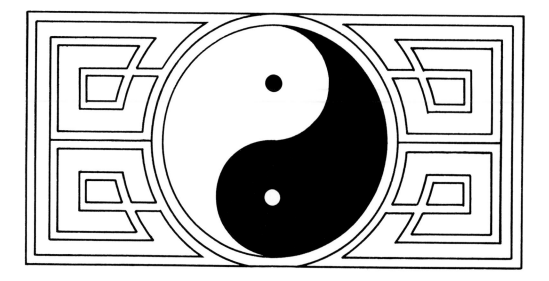

Now let's bring that understanding down to work in our own lives. First it is best to explore the characteristics of masculine and feminine energies at the universal level, and then see how they reflect at the human level. According to the *I-Ching, Yang,* or masculine energy, is creative, outgoing, and originates as heaven. *Yin*, the feminine energy, is receptive and yielding. It is pictured as the earth, as nature.

The earth is always looking towards heaven, looking towards God. It is how the feminine energy, the earth, the bearer of children, the Mother, is continually connected to God. She has the quality of devotion.

Heaven is always looking towards the earth. The man must look to the woman to find God. This is the image of how a man and a woman can realize their soul qualities. When we each learn the two parts of the dance we can always keep moving closer and closer to a harmonious life of balance and vitality.

One side of the dance is feminine. The feminine energy is space. It is receptive, child-bearing and nurturing. It is the sustainer of life. If we did not have a mother, a nurturer, we would not be able to survive. Mother is nature, mother is food. Mother is the earth and is responsible for everything that is in and on the earth. She is the bearer of life. To live we must have food and that food comes from the mother; originally from the mother's breast and then later from Mother Earth. We constantly need that nurturing energy in order to live.

Nurturing is giving. The woman knows how to give through her devotion and service. By nurturing her children, her husband, other people, plants, and animals, the

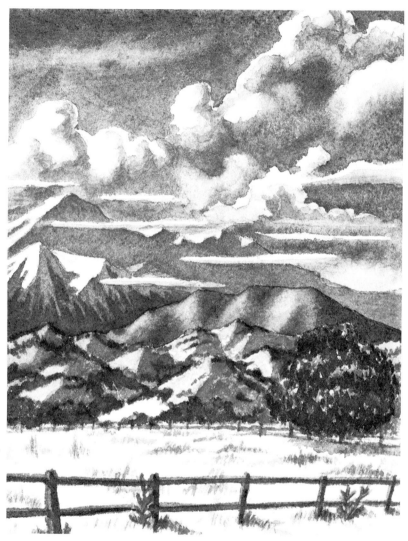

Heaven is the Creative, Earth is the Receptive.

woman is able to learn devotion. Giving food, while conscious that it is a blessing from the Lord, awakens her devotion to God. Each time she gives food she gives it up to God. Every woman possesses this ability. She thanks the power, thanks the God that is inside of her and everything that is around her. In this way the feminine quality of devotion emerges and grows.

The more we are able to accept our feminine quality, the more we will be able to accept our emotions and the emotions of those around us. The feminine is "water." The main quality of the earth is the ocean (water) and everything that lives in it. The ocean is constantly changing, going up and down with the tides. That movement and change is inside every woman in the form of her menstrual cycle, which is intimately linked to her emotions. That cycle provides for the continuation of life.

Just as the sun and moon affect the pull of the tides, they also affect the pull of the water within the woman. A woman has more water than a man physically, emotionally, and mentally. She can look at the moon and feel that pull inside herself. The magnetism is there.

The menstrual cycle is a graphic way for both men and women to understand each other. It is a method of dealing with the emotions, pain, and negativity in a positive form. Every month, if a woman has not conceived, nature provides her with a beautiful elimination system. She gets her period and releases a part of her that dies: the egg and the blood. She becomes more emotional and less conscious around that time period, and maybe even a little grumpy and crabby. It is an opportunity for her to get rid of all the toxins she has taken in during that month. For a husband and wife it also means she is eliminating all the man's negativity, emotions, and unconsciousness that she has absorbed in her intimacy with him. It is a golden opportunity for a man to get a reflection back of how emotional and unconscious he has been during that month.

When we come to understand that through this cycle the woman is in constant touch with the relationship of life and death, we can accept the feminine quality that is inside each one of us. That feminine quality is change, and within nature the only constant is change. This paradox is what the woman is all about.

During the menstrual period a woman can drink more fluids to assist the elimination of toxins from the body. She can also focus her emotions and have a good time doing something emotional and unconscious like arguing. This is where the man can help. Both partners can pick a time period and argue, get it all out, and yet still remember that it is all unconscious, emotional, and doesn't mean anything. Usually men get caught up in arguing with a woman at this time. They both take it all very seriously, hurt each other, and cry for a divorce.

Perhaps the man runs away from the emotions and disappears until it is all over. Usually he goes fishing or he goes drinking because he is still attracted to the water. Instead of running away from emotions, we can be grateful that nature has given us an opportunity to let go of negativity by working with the woman's cycle.

So, if we follow the entire cycle of the woman, we can learn about the ups and downs of emotion. The best way to follow this cycle is by studying the feminine production of the cervical mucus that controls whether the sperm reaches the egg. The mucus has fertile and infertile times which can be identified by various characteristics. Beginning right after her period, as she gets closer to the time of ovulation the woman builds up in consciousness. She is waxing like the moon. Just as the full moon totally reflects the light of the sun, so at her ovulation, the woman is the most receptive to the male energy. She is also the most creative at that time because she can conceive a child and therefore create new life.

If there is no conception, the waning time begins. The energy decreases as the time of the period draws near, and the woman becomes less and less conscious and more and more emotional. Finally, the time of the period arrives and an emotional, mental, and physical elimination happens. Menstruation is how nature keeps everything clean.

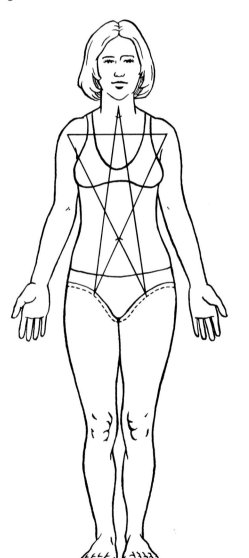

The Five-Pointed Star

The five-pointed star describes the feminine energy pattern in each individual. In a woman, the five-pointed star is the primary, dominant energy pattern. In a man, the five-pointed star is the secondary energy pattern.

This understanding of physical elimination also applies to morning sickness during pregnancy. Vomiting gets rid of all the toxins and keeps the diaphragm open to make room for the child. Nature simply pushes out the negativity.

We live in a world of negativity and stress. Our supermarkets, filled with dead food, reflect our disease. The food is frozen, canned, boxed, and wrapped. All nature is gone from it. Our food is lifeless. This makes us all feel like death ourselves, whether it's at a conscious or an unconscious level.

My feeling is, one reason women today are so angry is because they are serving dead food to the ones they love. The nurturing part of themselves has been denied life. This constant denial is one reason breast cancer is rampant in the United States today, occurring in one out of every five women. The breasts, the symbol as well as the actual physical manifestation of the feminine quality of nurturing, are rotting away by the age of thirty. We are now in the death-throes of this feminine quality. Women are out of balance and that is when a disease situation occurs.

Now the other side of the dance is the masculine energy. Men are having the same difficulty as women manifesting a healthy primary energy. When the male energy is in balance it is like heaven. It is creative, strong, outgoing, and directive. It has authority in its knowledge. There are two types of knowledge. One is intellectual knowing and the other is intuitive; that is, being able to perceive the subtle qualities of the people and events around us. The authority of balanced male energy gives a person a sense of direction. When masculine energy has that sense of direction, it needs to be responsible when expressing it. Responsibility is a main attribute of the male energy.

Traditionally, it has been said a man is a real man if he is true to his word. Then he is honorable. If a man is committed to his word he is a man of God. If a man does not take responsibility for his primary energy, then he loses his backbone and we call him spineless. This understanding sheds some light on why we are seeing so much back trouble in the United States today. Neither men nor women are taking full responsibility for their primary energy.

An even bigger problem for men today is heart attacks. The heart is one of the main muscles in the body. In general, men have bulkier muscles than women. When the heart pumps it creates a rhythmic beat. There are no harmonics in it as in the up and down cycle of a woman. When a man is healthy and in balance with his male energy, that rhythm will be steady. When the rhythm of the male energy is off and jerky, running and stopping, disease attacks the heart. We are now experiencing a national epidemic of unbalanced male energy and heart disease is the greatest symptom.

Male energy, as expressed in the *I-Ching*, is creativity. Creativity is productive action and with action comes the responsibility for what we create. Most people misunderstand the creative aspect of male energy. Real creativity demands vulnerability. When we become truly creative, we make ourselves vulnerable to other people. This concept is particularly obvious with artists because they go through a lot of pain showing their work. They have to make themselves vulnerable in the position of creativity. So a man in balance will be very vulnerable through his creativity. He expresses himself, exposes himself, and is trustworthy.

When we are able to accept our masculine energy and our word is true, then we are responsible. When our crea-

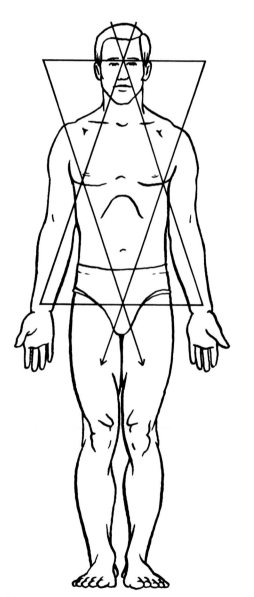

The Six-Pointed Star
The six-pointed star describes the masculine energy pattern in each individual. In a man, the six-pointed star is the primary, dominant energy pattern. In a woman, the six-pointed star is the secondary energy pattern.

tive selves become vulnerable, and we expose ourselves and everything we do, then another paradox occurs. We become so strongly creative and masculine that we manifest our feminine energy of vulnerability and devotion. We become nurturing. We are able to recognize and accept our emotions.

This healthy male energy perfectly complements the woman's situation. To be a healthy woman we must be devotional, nurturing, and giving. We manifest vulnerability and we have no secrets. Our words are truth. Then we become creative and responsible. Our energies are in a complementary balance, which gives us great vitality and harmony.

In the *I-Ching* this transformation is illustrated when a line of a hexagram is called a "changing line," which means it becomes so strongly and completely masculine or feminine, it changes into the other. Each side has that potential within it; the seed of the other. When our masculine and feminine sides work together in harmony, then we can be men and women in the fullest sense of the words.

Learning about the attributes of the masculine and feminine energies is a tool for looking at ourselves and the polarity of the unconscious, emotional reactions that are occurring within and around us. Once we know who we are, then we can look at ourselves in relation to the soul and the living light that surrounds us. This is how as individuals we can learn from this school we live in called Mother Earth.

What I am sharing is not a sexist understanding. Today women are so concerned with power. What I am teaching is that women have the greater power when they are truly receptive. Then they are the foundation of life. They are looking directly at God and feeling that devotion. Actually, this is the case for both women and men when they manifest true receptivity. In receptivity is tremendous power.

For our own healing process it is vital that we don't get caught in the role play of, "I should do this," and "I should not do that." Let's begin to develop our primary energy. Once we do that, the other side takes care of itself. The balance happens automatically.

What I'm talking about is really not role playing at all. It is understanding the male and female qualities inside ourselves and learning how to flow with that natural energy. For a woman, each man is a reflection of the male quality within herself, whether he is a husband, a father, a brother, or a son. For a man, any woman resonates with, and reflects back, the feminine energy within himself.

As soon as we say men must do this and women must do that, we are dividing men and women and also dividing ourselves. This is hurtful and destructive to the healing process. Learning how to know ourselves by concentrating and going within becomes impossible. So the key here is to be flexible. Flexibility is a feminine quality whether it is exhibited by a woman or a man who is expressing the feminine energy. The feminine energy of the universe is giving, in terms of both nurturing and yielding.

Feminine stability comes within "form," just as the ocean is defined by land. To use another example, the tree has roots that go deep into the earth. The tree, which is a form, is able to live a long time and grow strong because it can bend in the wind. The roots have gone so deep that

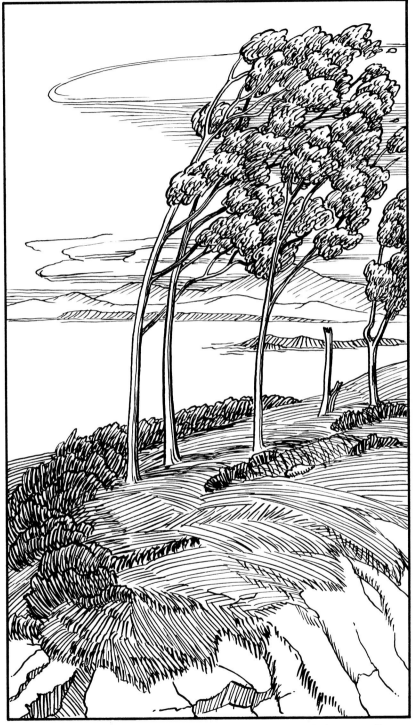

Trees bending in the wind display the feminine quality
of yielding, the power of flexibility.

the tree is able to withstand the pressure of a hurricane by giving, yielding, and being flexible. It's the same principle with a pregnant woman. Her body gives in many different ways in order to accommodate a child. A man catching a football yields to the ball so it does not bounce off his hands.

When the feminine energy becomes rigid it gets cancer. It loses its motion. This is symbolized by a lake when it loses its movement and the water becomes stagnant. The lake becomes a cesspool and all life in it dies. So form, the feminine energy, must have motion, life, and flexibility. When we lose our flexibility we lose our vitality. Another national epidemic is unbalanced female energy, the great symptom being cancer.

Healing occurs when the relationship of our male and female energy is in harmony. Once again, it comes down to accepting what we are: the masculine and feminine, the positive and negative qualities. When we can accept both, then we can let go and learn from the mistakes we have made. That is what life is all about. We are not really living unless we are making mistakes. If we repeat the same mistakes, then we are killing ourselves. We experience premature death when we repeat our mistakes.

When we become conscious of energy and life within form, we are able to understand the soul and how the soul lives and functions in this world. To have this awareness means being in the present. When we are fully in the present, we are taking responsibility for our present actions which sow the seeds for our future. Then we can take full responsibility for our past deeds and see how they created our present.

Because the soul is conscious it continues to move in the direction of good. As we become more conscious we create more good. What is so beautiful about being alive with polarity is accepting that emotions are mechanical, and then learning how to move out of that mechanical part of ourselves. By accepting our emotions, accepting what is happening now, we are able to become conscious.

Doing this, we can take a step back and observe ourselves. We can watch our minds and our emotional reactions. Actually, we like to be mechanical. I picture our minds as people watching a tennis match. Their heads just go back and forth. One side of the mind hits the other side of the mind and the reacting energy continues to bounce back and forth. It's madness.

Taking that step back is really all we can do. As human beings we need to be the observer. We must not claim what we observe as our own. Our knowledge is not our own and neither is the whirlwind of feelings, emotions, and reactions that are around and inside us. By not claiming them as our own, we can then be with people in consciousness. We can be with nature and live with nature. We can live with the Power. We can live with God. And most important of all, we can live with ourselves.

II

Our Journey Into Creation

The physical body is a crystallization of the mind and is formed by the emotions. The emotions are what actually create the physical body, which means the mind is the emotions which *are* the physical body. The body is a map. It is a physical manifestation of our destiny. We are, right now, in the way we look, the type of face we have, our nose, our mouth, our feet and our toes—everything about us, a map of our whole destiny. We can tell the type of animals we were, the type of plants we were, and the kind of human beings we have been in our past lives, by the mapping of our physical body.

Our destiny is the result of our *karma*: our present situation in life that has come as a result of all the past actions that we have created in past associations and past relationships. Our destiny has been created over eons of time; it is automatically recorded. The Akashic Record (see Glossary) starts with our original sin, the original action on this earth for each of us, and continues to record every action from that time on. Each action then creates a reaction and that energy manifests into lifetimes of events that happen over and over again.

We cannot change our destiny. What we can do is exercise our free will, which is the attitude we adopt towards the events that come to us. We can choose to be either positive or negative as our karmas come back to us, as our destiny unfolds. What is past is past. What we can do now is choose to be more conscious of our actions in the present so we create a more positive future.

Acting positively means we raise our own vibration so the reactions we experience, our own reactions and the reactions of others to us, do not come back negatively. When we have a high vibration, it means we are in harmony with the universe because our actions have become more pure and more positive. Thus, the reactions in our life will reflect that positivity. So it is actually the attitude we choose that constitutes our free will. It is our attitude that helps our soul gain its freedom from the physical world and the endless wheel of birth and death.

Our soul is imprisoned by the mind when it is in the physical body. The mind has the power because it is made up of actions and reactions: all our karmas that we have already created. The mind is much more powerful than the soul when they are knotted together in the physical body because the mind is in its own domain at this level. In other words, the mind is dominant on the physical plane. And yet, the mind is not everything. There is still the soul, there is still the energy. Without the soul or the life force we would not exist. What we need to understand is that the mind is not the soul.

Most of us think that the mind is what is giving us all these thoughts, making us run smoothly, making us tick, so to speak. In actuality, the soul itself is the energizer and that soul energy is what is activating the mind. Now there are many different words for the energy itself. Some people call it God, other people call it Light or Sound, while others call it Love. Right now, my best description of it, as a Westerner, is the electricity in the wall socket that keeps the tape recorder going.

Our mind is very much a tape recorder. It records all of our actions and all of our thoughts. We can see that quality we have, of being like a tape recorder, as we watch ourselves act and react. We just keep repeating the same things over and over again. It's like the groove of a record when the needle gets caught. The needle, like the mind, repeats the same groove over and over and over.

It takes a major event to switch the groove on our record. When that event occurs, the soul energy begins to pull us. We are not in control of the pull which moves us from one groove of the record to another. Anytime we are seeking a better attitude, it is the soul that is pulling us. The Lord is pulling us anytime we are doing anything positive: like therapy, for instance. At the same time, the grace of this pull toward the positive is written into our destiny, a result of past actions and choices.

Our soul is a reflection of the One. It is a particle of the Life. God is Life. So this particle of God, of the One, is trapped in this human form. Somewhere along the line, as we become more conscious, we start to get pulled. The soul starts to get pulled because the soul is who we truly

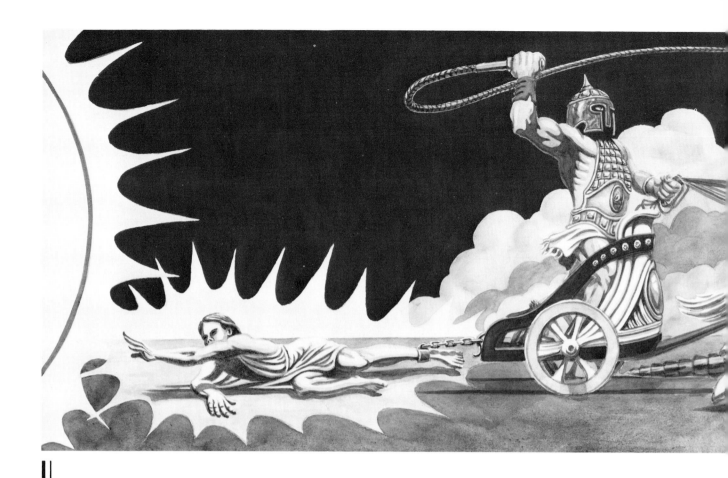

are. The soul begins to get free. If the soul had its way, it
would burn this body right up and just take off to reunite
with its Source. The mind does not want to let go of the
soul because the mind enjoys the pleasures of the world.
The mind is in control on this earthly plane, even though,
paradoxically, the mind is actually being activated by the
soul.

There are two aspects of mind: the complex and the
simple, the intellectual and the intuitive. The complex,
intellectual side is our rational mind. It is the part of
ourselves that needs proof and tends to reject anything
that is not tangible or scientific. The simple side is intuitive. This side is our animal nature. We tend to get stuck
with our intuitive feelings and perceptions. We see visions

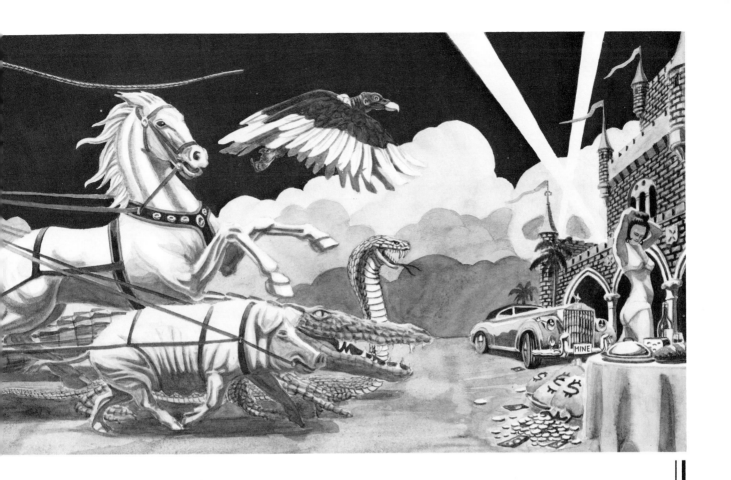

The Soul's Dilemma

This is an allegorical painting of the soul longing for its Source. The soul is chained to the mind which is in turn pulled by the senses into the material world. The soul is portrayed as an innocent youth, reaching toward the Light that is radiating from the Lord. The intellectual aspect of the mind is shown by the chariot and driver. The mind is mechanical, running in familiar grooves. It wields the whip of karma or justice and dominates the soul. The emotional part of the mind is portrayed by animals. The horse is *pride:* stiff-necked, unruly, "above it all." The sow is *greed:* gluttonous, pig-headed, selfish. The crocodile is *lust:* steely-eyed, thick-skinned, and unfeeling. The snake is *anger:* quickly aroused and striking out without forethought. The vulture is *attachment* to the lifeless, outward aspects of people and things. Sensual pleasure, wealth, and fantasy lure the mind as death lurks in the background.

and think we are seeing God. This is nonsense. The animals have intuition. Intuition, like intellect, is still Mind. It is not spiritual.

By accepting and understanding the nature of mind, we can get to the soul. Mind is dense. We have got to go through the mind, this denseness, to get to the soul. The only power the soul has in the body is its power to give us an understanding of how the mind works, until the soul pulls us out of the body and through the mind itself. Then the mind becomes our friend. At that point the mind no longer has any duality. There is no more reaction. We will be free of any good karma or bad karma. All of our karmas will be burned. Our sins will be washed away. At that moment the soul is free. It is no longer chained to the body or mind.

On the other hand, we need a body to communicate with each other as souls. For this communication to happen we need to use our mind, the original blueprint for whatever we do. The power in the blueprint stems from all the past actions we have created, the essence of mind. The blueprint originates from the sameness we all share which we call Universal Mind. Universal Mind is still Mind. It's just that it's so much more powerful than the individual mind, we tend to confuse it with the soul. The soul has no blueprint. The soul is the Life. The soul is what enables the blueprint to exist.

This original blueprint of our mind, which is fixed by all our past karmas, is what determines the kind of body we are going to have in this life. It is as if the soul is an architect and in attempting to build its house, its temple of the Lord, it creates a blueprint, an idea of what the house will be. That idea is the mind.

The body that our soul enters is a reflection of the mind which is an accumulation of all our past actions. The soul says, "Okay, you've done these specific things in your other lifetimes on earth and now you are going to learn this, this and this because you didn't learn these things before. This time, your body is going to be shaped this way because of the things you've done and been in the past."

So, the first aspect of the mind is the blueprint. From that blueprint the soul brings down the energy into the physical. Bringing the energy down into the physical means that the energy gets slowed down and transformed. It gets pulled down further and further from the Source. The energy divides and divides into greater and greater polarity until we become the gross physical body. This body is our vehicle from the One, our gift from God, that allows us to learn our lessons, pay off our karmic debts, and balance our karmas through emotional attraction and attachment to other people and things. This body is our human birth.

This understanding is pretty foreign to the Western mind because what we are talking about is reincarnation. We reincarnate by the mind reproducing itself over and over and over. Our original blueprint repeats itself over and over from parent to parent: father, mother, mother, father, and all the parents we have ever come from. Then we pass on these patterns to our children. We live and we die and we live and we die, passing on our blueprint, our ideas and our mental patterns, from one generation to another.

We reincarnate because of our attachments. Attachment is what allows the mind to reproduce itself. We copy and mimic. We have done this ever since the original conception. We have copied and imprinted exactly what was imprinted on our parents' mind at the time they conceived us, and that imprint keeps getting passed on. It is our attachment to each set of parents, those particular people, that keeps us coming back into this world of birth and death, pleasure and pain: this world of duality, of polarity.

We come into this world as a reaction. Conception is a reaction to the union of the sperm of our father with the egg of our mother. An incredible reaction takes place when the sperm and the egg merge, and it is from this reaction that we are created. Following our blueprint, the cells just keep on growing and growing and growing. They keep reproducing until a whole human being is formed. I think of this reaction, of conception, as being much more powerful than any atomic bomb that we could create.

The emotional relationship that we inherit from the past, the experiences that our parents were going through until the exact moment of conception, reproduce over and over for the entire life of the child. That emotional make-up defines the entire blueprint until the person dies. In other words, the whole building process does not come to an end until we die. The last lesson we go through is death.

Everything that we have not yet realized in ourselves, everything we have not yet learned about ourselves and our passions, comes in with our soul at the moment of conception, through the emotional attachment we have to

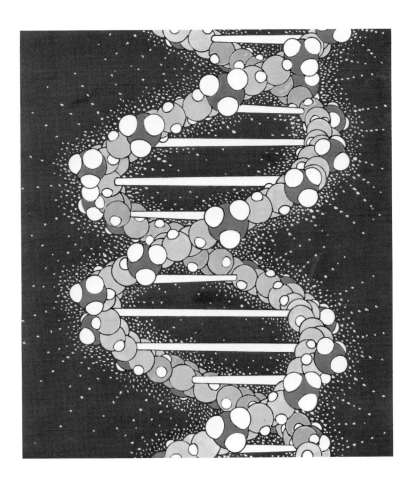

DNA, found in the central core (nucleus) of every cell in the body, is the physical counterpart of our mental blueprint. Mental patterns may have an intimate connection to the gene sequence patterns in the DNA molecule. If we remember that the solid-looking atoms pictured here are actually little clouds of energy, we can begin to perceive the solid forms around us as energy patterns. We can also see how our bodies are a physical mapping of the combined mental energy patterns of our parents.

our parents and their attachment to us. The lessons continue to repeat themselves until we die. Every breath we take, every expression we make, has already been laid out for us. The lessons have already been mapped, and that mapping starts at the moment of conception, at that reaction. The mapping of our destiny unfolds from the first breath we take when we are born until the last breath we take when we die.

We come into this world alone and we leave alone. We come into the world as a soul: as an individual with already established past associations with other souls, other people, other thoughts, and other attitudes. Then we attach with those thoughts and attitudes to two people who have the exact same attitudes, the exact same thoughts as we do: our parents. Those thoughts and attitudes then get crystallized as the original energy moves down. The physical body is gradually woven in this way during the nine-month period from conception to birth. This development of a new human being begins the story of how karma gets worked out through emotional attraction in the physical body.

In order for us to understand energy and how it works we need to go back to the Source. The original energy first starts out as One. This One energy can be called God, the Lord, or the One. A particle of the Lord steps down from the spiritual realm into the mental realm of the mind. As soon as it steps down into the mind this particle of the Lord splits. It creates three main energies: fire, air, and water. As this energy descends further into the creation, it slows down in vibration and crystallizes until it becomes the physical body.

This concept of energy we are dealing with uses the three energy principles of fire, air, and water, because when we move into the world we are no longer One. We are not totally the Lord. We have a soul which is a particle of the Lord, but it is not the total energy. Energy can mean God, the Lord, or the Source. We can call this energy any name we want. The name is not important because this energy is the essence of Oneness, it is where there is no pain. None. Zero! One way we can know that we are in the world is that we feel pain. As soon as we have pain these three basic principles are functioning.

The first principle is the fire principle. It is outgoing. It is the creative energy that shoots us into this earthly

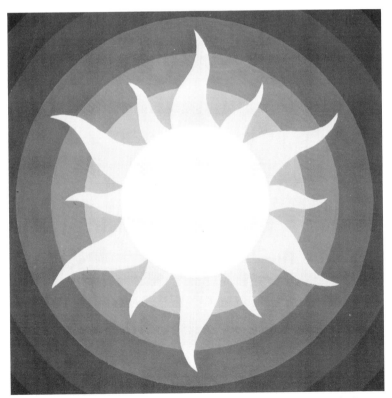

The sun, the symbol of the fiery, creative principle.

realm. We can see it at work at the time of birth when the womb opens up and the baby comes shooting out; the fiery principle is that explosion. It is the fire of the sun. If we did not have the sun, souls could not exist on this planet. The fiery energy is the outgoing, creative, masculine energy. It is what creates the muscles in the body. Warmth and fire are the fiery principle of creativity.

Both men and women have this energy. All of creation has this energy. We cannot call it our own; it is only differentiated now because we are not One anymore. We have split from the Oneness, into this world, and created this mind, which later created this body.

The second energy we have is the water principle. The water principle is all of our form. It is the body we have and it is anything that creates form. It is also the earth because out of the water comes the earth. The water energy crystallizes into forms like the earth. The watery principle is the feminine, receptive energy. For example, when the sky is blue and we look into the water, the water is blue. When the sky is grey, the water is grey. The water is totally reflective. The water is the reflecting, receptive energy to the creative.

This receptive water principle can be seen in the cycles of life, the ups and downs of life. It is in the tide as it is pulled back and forth by the attraction of the sun and moon, by that power, by that gravity. The water principle is that pulling, that magnetism. It is the basis of our earthly emotions. These emotions make up our unconscious mind and they come from the watery principle, whereas the conscious part of our mind is the creative, fire principle.

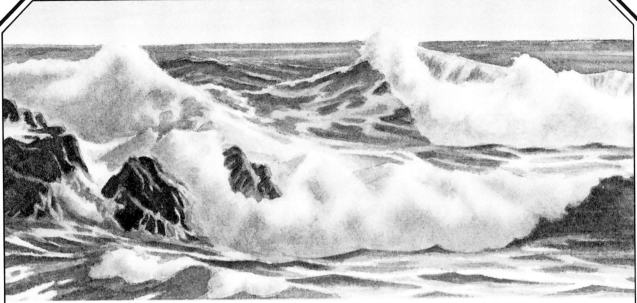

The ocean, the symbol of the watery, receptive principle.

When we are receptive, we are eliminative. This receptivity is the aspect of ourselves that is able to eliminate the toxins from our bodies and minds. When we are receptive we are eliminative because we have to be clear in order to be receptive. We have to be a totally shining mirror to reflect what is coming to us.

One of the problems we have today is that we do not recognize, or even know, what receptivity really is; receptivity is pure reflection. Calm, pure water is reflective and that reflection is the essence of the feminine energy within our body-mind.

So now we have two main energies. We have the fiery principle which is the masculine, and we have the watery principle which is the feminine. As the energy splits from the One, it still retains a reflection of itself. This reflection of the One is the air principle. It is the third main energy after the split. The airy principle is that part of the air which is essential to life. It is that first breath we take when we come into this world. The airy energy is what the

Eastern Indians and the Vedas call *prana*. Some people call it the life-force. It allows life to exist and allows us to breathe. It allows the fish to have their fun swimming around in the water. We could not have the creative fire, or the receptive water, without this air, without this life-force.

The airy principle is the balance point. It is the point where neither the creative nor the receptive is dominant. It is totally balanced. This airy energy is the *Wu-Wei* of the Taoists, the effortless effort. It is when suddenly, for a

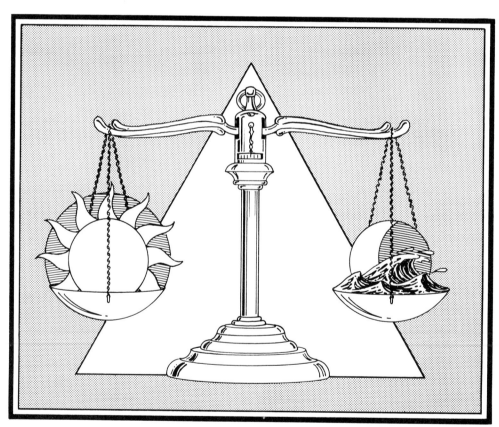

The air principle is the neutral balance point between the fire principle and the water principle. The scales represent neutrality, balance, and perfect justice in this world of polarities.

moment, we are able to recognize our soul, when we are in total harmony and balance with the universe. It is when we are separate and yet still able to catch a glimpse of our Oneness with the Divine. It happens when we have stepped out of the way and allowed the energy to take over.

When we come to that point of recognition, when we glimpse our Oneness, we have achieved what I call the Trinity; the triune function, which is the balance of the three main energies we have in the universe. We can call these three main energies by many names. By whatever names we choose, they still make up the main triangle that serves as the foundation of the physical creation. They can be called: Fire-Air-Water, Masculine-Neuter-Feminine, *Raja-Sattva-Tamas*, and Action-Nothing-Reaction, to name a few.

Now this is not pure spirit we are talking about. This is how spirit comes down into mind and starts to create the body. The mind is the formative, blueprint stage in the process of transmuting the essence of spirit into the substance of matter. The body is the dense matter of the mind. The soul descends into the creation and creates the original sin, the original action, and everything stems from that moment. If we have an action, then we have to have a reaction, and that's it. It is a law of physics, of creation. Then we have a mind. Before that we did not have a mind.

As soon as the soul moves out of the spirit realm and into the mental realm, density creates a reaction, because everything here is a reaction. It is like a waterfall, for example. The soul is not feeling any influence of the mind until it takes that one step into the waterfall. At that moment, suddenly the soul is deluged. From that time on, it is just reaction piled on top of reaction. However, if the soul moved a half an inch away from the waterfall, the actions and reactions would not have an effect on the soul.

So, as we trace the journey of the soul downwards into the creation, the soul steps down from the One and splits

CHART of EQUIVALENTS

Source = God   = Spiritual = Energy =   One

Nothing = Sattva =   Mental   =   Air   = Three Principles
                     (causal)

Action = Raja = Emotional = Fire = Five Elements
                     (astral)

Reaction = Tamas = Physical = Water = Twenty-Five Combinations

Arrows show the descent of the One Energy into matter. Crystallization of energy increases with its distance from the source.

into the three original vibrations, which are action, reaction, and the moment in between, which is no action, no anything, nothing. Anytime we have something on either pole there has to be something in the middle, even if it is nothing.

Here in the mental realm exists the highest vibration of form. It is here, at the causal level, that we experience the original blueprint of the mind. The essence of our mind, which is made up of all our past actions, manifests at the causal level in terms of five *ideas*. These five ideas are the vibrations or essences of the five elements of earth, water, fire, air, and ether. These five ideas, at the causal level, are the result of the stepdown of energy of the three principles of air, fire, and water, from the spiritual realm into the mental realm.

From the causal level, the energy steps down once again to the astral level where the ideas of the original blueprint become *action*. The five earthly emotions first begin to manifest at the astral level. These five emotions correspond to each one of the five elements. Earth is fear, water is attachment, fire is anger, air is desire, and ether is grief. In the mother's womb, where the child is still connected to the astral, these five emotions interweave into twenty-five combinations and create the physical body, the *reaction*.

So let's re-trace this chain of events back upwards. The physical body, at the physical level, is the reaction. It is the Tamas, the water principle. It is the reaction to the action of the five emotions at the astral level: the Raja, the fire principle. These five emotions are the action, the stepdown from the ideas at the causal level: the Sattva, the air

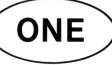

ONE

The 3 principles of Air, Fire, and Water govern the stepdown of energy from the Spiritual to the Physical level.

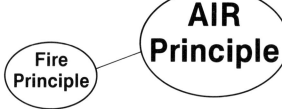

AIR Principle

Fire Principle

Water Principle

IDEAS of the 5 elements

(Space) (Air) (Fire) (Water) (Earth)

SATTVA or CAUSAL LEVEL

Air Principle dominating

Ideas or essences of the five elements begin here.

FIRE Principle

Air Principle

Water Principle

ACTION of the 5 elements

Space Air Fire Water Earth

RAJA or ASTRAL LEVEL

Fire Principle dominating

Action of the five elements begins here.

Air Principle

Fire Principle

WATER Principle

REACTIONS of the 5 elements

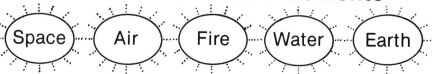

Space Air Fire Water Earth

This is the level of emotion (e-motion: from Latin — to move out i.e., into the world).

TAMAS or PHYSICAL LEVEL

Water Principle dominating

Reactions and crystallization of the five elements begin here.

principle. This chain represents the relationship of the principles and the elements and how, as energy, they crystallize into the human body.

In the physical body we experience life as an interplay of all three principles. We experience the five elements as physical form. Yet, in the Sattva, the air, is the highest understanding and the key to all life. The qualities of the air principle are also the qualities of higher consciousness: the observer, neutral, beyond action and reaction. There is tremendous power here, the power that sustains all creation. As we become more conscious, we experience this power more and more fully.

The final stepdown of the emotions is the actual weaving of the body within the womb at the physical level. On an energy level, this happens when these five emotional vibrations interact. Making the body is like mixing ingredients in a recipe. The body is a product of the actual mixing of the different elements: ether, air, fire, water, and earth. This mixing produces the earthly emotions of grief, desire, anger, attachment (love), and fear. These emotions then interact to create our bones, our hair, our flesh, and our blood. The force that creates these emotions within the womb is the original attachment of our parents, the emotional magnetism that brought them together to create a child.

At each level of the stepdown, from the pure spiritual to the physical plane, there is one principle of the original three that is dominant. At the causal level, which is the original blueprint where the five elements are present only as ideas, the airy principle is dominant. On the astral level, where the emotions are first developed, the fiery

Physical Level or Tamas
Where the emotions actually form the physical body

This chart shows the interactions or reactions of the 5 elements and the 25 products of their combinations.

5th Chakra — Ether or Space

Emotions are created within the 5th chakra by the combination of ether with the other elements.

Elements	Negative Aspects	Positive Aspects
Ether + Ether =	Grief	Nothing or Longing
Ether + Air =	Desire	Selflessness
Ether + Fire =	Anger	Power or Warmth
Ether + Water =	Attachment	Continence
Ether + Earth =	Fear	Courage

These five emotions interact within the four lower chakras to weave the body and create its functions. They combine as follows:

4th Chakra **AIR** **DESIRE** 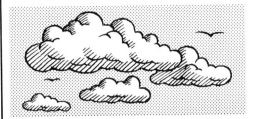	+ Desire	= Speed
	+ Grief	= Lengthening
	+ Anger	= Shaking
	+ Attachment	= Movement
	+ Fear	= Contraction

3rd Chakra **FIRE** **ANGER** 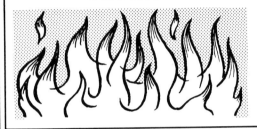	+ Anger	= Hunger
	+ Grief	= Sleep
	+ Desire	= Thirst
	+ Attachment	= Luster
	+ Fear	= Laziness

2nd Chakra **WATER** **ATTACHMENT** 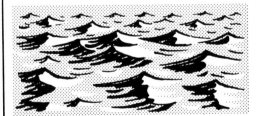	+ Attachment	= Semen/Egg
	+ Grief	= Saliva
	+ Desire	= Sweat
	+ Anger	= Urine
	+ Fear	= Blood

1st Chakra **EARTH** **FEAR** 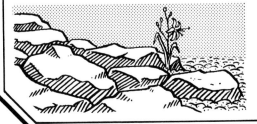	+ Fear	= Bones
	+ Grief	= Hair
	+ Desire	= Skin
	+ Anger	= Blood Vessels
	+ Attachment	= Flesh

principle is dominant. The physical level of matter is dominated by the watery principle.

So the emotions are developed within the womb at the moment of conception, as the creative energy of the sperm interacts with the receptive energy of the egg. The union of the fire and the water creates a balance between the two which is the air. It is through the air that the soul can enter the womb and inhabit a physical body. Through the reaction of the conception, the law of physics takes off, all the cells start dividing, and life begins to emerge in a physical form.

What I want to share at this point is that out of the basic three principles come the five elements that create the physical body, vibrationally, through the emotions. The creation of the human form happens in the womb, within the ether, which is the center of the emotions on the physical plane.

Even though the emotions are physical, they are not tangible like the rest of the body. We cannot grab hold of them. The physical embodiment of the emotions, the ether, is the highest of the physical manifestations in creation. When a child is in the womb, even though it is within the etheric energy, it is connected to another plane of existence. It is in the astral region. There are seven chakras, or energy centers, in the body. The top two are spiritual and mental, not physical. The ether chakra is the highest of the remaining five physical chakras.

So, the ether is the ruler of the emotions in the physical. The emotions are created within the etheric energy in the womb, through the interaction of the five elements, with the dominant element being the ether. Half of the

The Ether Chakra

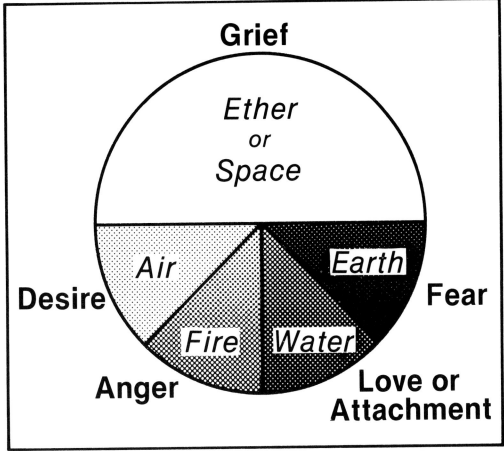

The emotions are produced by the combination of
the dominant element of ether with the four
other elements of air, fire, water, and earth.

original essence of each element remains dominant in the astral region. The second half divides into four equal parts, preparing for the interaction that will take place at the physical level. For example, when the whole vibration of ether steps down into the physical, one half of it, the dominant element of ether, interacts with the other half, the remaining four elements of air, fire, water, and earth.

The main quality of the ether is the emotion of grief, a feeling of nothingness. The emotion of desire is produced by the interaction of air and the dominant element of ether. The emotion of anger is the product of the dominant element of ether with fire. The emotion of attachment (love) is the product of water combining with the dominant element of ether. Fear is produced by the combination of earth with the dominant element of ether.

Each emotion creates a chakra, an energy center within the body, from which each emotion radiates physical manifestations. Ether, the highest of the five, is located at the throat. Desire (from the air) is in the chest. Anger (from the fire) is located in the solar plexus. Attachment, or love, (from the water) is situated in the pelvis, and fear (from the earth) is located near the base of the spine, in the area of the rectum. These earthly emotions are a physical form of the five original elements or ideas at the causal level: the original blueprint of our mind. First we have the emotions and out of the emotions come our physical bodies.

It is the emotions that draw our mother and father together. We call it magnetism. It is a pull, an attraction. After all, we're funny looking people. We have breasts and eyes, pelvises and genitals. Our bodies are actually very strange and not very attractive when we look at them objectively, as an observer. It is our emotions that are attractive. Emotions are what pull us to one another. That pull is unconscious. We are not aware of it. That magnetism, that pull of the emotions, is what brings a man and woman together to have a relationship. Emotional attraction, or what we call love, is an unconscious reaction. It is "what makes the world go round." At conception, we are bringing together emotionally the masculine and feminine energies so the soul can start to merge into the body that is being created.

What makes human beings different from plants and animals is that we have the consciousness to be able to understand our emotions. We are not unconscious. We are not totally at the whim of our emotions. Animals have emotions. Emotions are unconscious; they just automatically happen. Human beings have both sides: the unconscious and the conscious.

When a tiger goes to kill, to get its meat, it is emotional. The tiger kills for its food because it is hungry. Human beings have the ability to understand their emotions and they are able to bring that understanding to consciousness. If, instead of being ruled totally by reaction, we human beings learn that our emotions are unconscious and reactionary, then we are able to switch, be more conscious, and take responsibility for being the highest form of life in this creation.

III

Understanding Positive and Negative Emotions:
Our Personalities and Our Diseases

The essence of Alive Polarity is the process of working with the five earthly emotions on a physical and psychological level to raise our consciousness so a healing phase can begin in our lives. By working with these emotions we are able to develop our awareness and understand how these emotions create the human body. We see how the emotional patterns that we absorbed from our parents affect our body-mind for the rest of our lives. We become more focused, and what naturally follows from this focus is a refinement of our vibration and a growth in our understanding. This work with the emotions is a spiralling process, a gradual upward movement. This process is our quest. From it we learn the way out of our human predicament.

The more imbalance we have with our emotions, the more disease we will have in our body. If the emotions are not "at ease," then the body will reflect that discomfort. The physical problem begins with the emotional imbalance. The emotion will create the problem. In order to understand diseases, we need to first understand how the emotions step down from the ether and create our entire physical make-up.

So let's explore the nature of the five emotions of grief, desire, anger, attachment (love), and fear. It is important to recognize that these five emotions are the physical step-down of the five elements that started at the causal level with the original blueprint of the mind. In other words, the emotions are the elements.

The first physical stepdown of the five elements occurs within the womb, in the ether. The ether is the highest physical manifestation. Through the interaction of the dominant element of ether with the four other elements, this fifth (ether) chakra combines to produce the five earthly emotions. The ether chakra is located at the throat.

Ether is the feminine quality of space. It is the space all around us, the space we feel outside and inside. It is the main feeling we have deep down. We think we are muscles, blood, and bones. We think we are emotions. In actuality, we are space. We are nothing. The main quality of space is nothing, no-thing. So when we are really in balance in our emotions, we will feel nothing. We will be attached to nothing. We will be nothing. We will be the observer. All that we see and feel, we will not be it, any of it. We will be no-thing. This is what I mean by space.

The first emotion from the ether element, that is created within the womb, is grief. The main quality of the ether (space) is actually grief or longing. When we are experiencing our space, that feeling of nothingness or emptiness, the highest vibration of that space is grief or longing

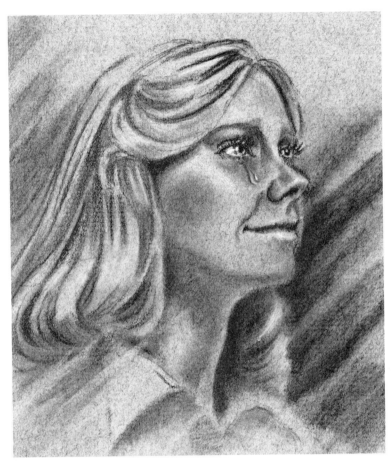

The positive aspect of grief is longing for the Lord.

for God. When we feel this longing, we are the most receptive to our higher self, or soul. Our emotions are being pulled toward our soul quality. The temple is then longing for the vibration of the Lord to fill the emptiness or space.

Each emotion has a positive and negative aspect. The positive aspect of the grief is feeling the space and then directing that feeling toward longing for the Lord. Suddenly, in feeling that space, we sense that being a human being is nothing. We are not like the animals. They are a part of us, but we are not animals. And we are not the

Lord, either. We recognize our separation from Him and feel our aloneness. We are neither the animal part of ourselves, or the God part, the soul. We are both and neither one, totally. So the positive aspect of grief is longing for the Lord: longing to be "That," and knowing we are not.

The negative side of grief is the "poor-me." This negative attitude, when we are in our grief, is non-acceptance of

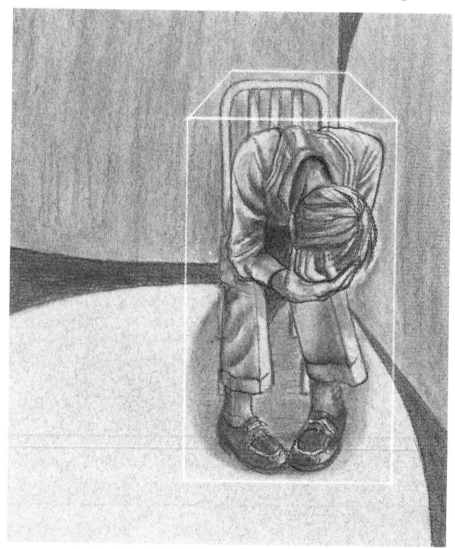

The negative aspect of grief is the "poor-me,"
feeling sorry for ourselves and our situation in life
which is the result of all our past actions.

the lessons that we have been given to learn and resentment toward God for putting us in particular situations. The "poor-me" happens when we will not take responsibility for the situations we have created by our past actions. A "poor-me" does not understand that we reap the fruit of the seeds we have sown, that we create all our own predicaments.

So, when we negatively experience the nothingness, the space that is around us, we end up feeling very sorry for ourselves that we are alone. In most situations when we come to the realization of our aloneness, we run. We feel, "Oh, poor-me, I have nothing. I am nobody." Then our grief is selfish. As a result, the negative emotion starts to physically affect the rest of our body. Other negative emotions are stirred up and the physical body becomes diseased.

The second emotion developed in the ether, within the womb, is desire. Desire results from the interaction of the dominant element of ether (space) with air. The positive aspect of desire is desiring God; desire for the perfection that we know is within each one of us, desire for the grace of God and the purity of the soul. We must have the desire in order to be pulled by our emotions upward to the Lord. Desire for the perfection of God is the positive aspect of desire.

The negative aspect of desire is the obsessive desire we all have experienced for the material things of this world. We constantly want more things. We feel the emptiness, the space, and we want to fill it with things and attachments to objects or people. Instead of seeking humility for the soul, we desire things. We fill up, instead of feeling the empti-

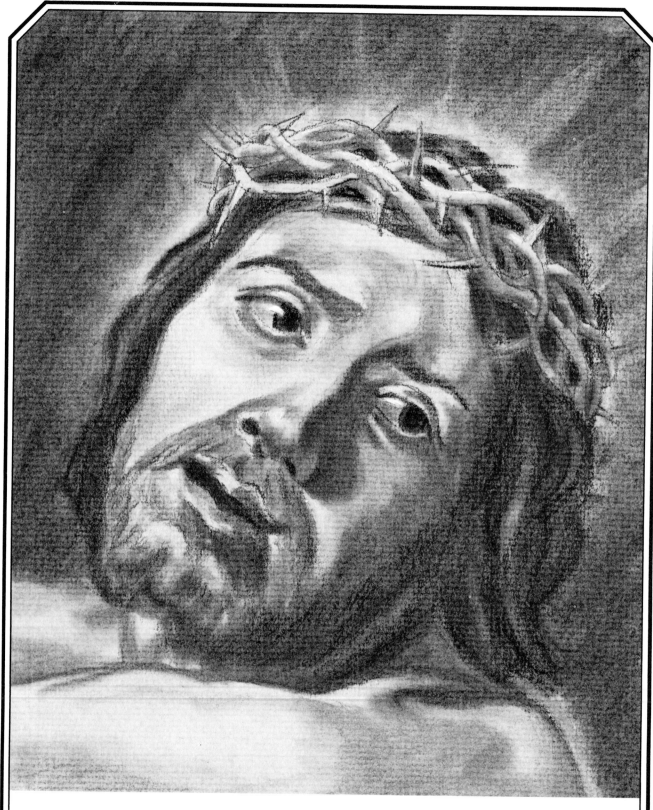

Christ, in His desire to do the Will of the Father and to be reunited with Him, is an example of positive desire. (After a painting by Velasquez.)

ness, instead of feeling the pain of the longing for reuniting with God.

The next emotion, anger, is created through the interaction of the dominant element of ether (space) with the fire element. The positive aspect of anger is its power and force. It is positive to be angry at the negative part of ourselves. That negativity is the part of our mind that refuses to look at the Lord and will get angry at other people instead. That anger is guilt. We are guilty about a number

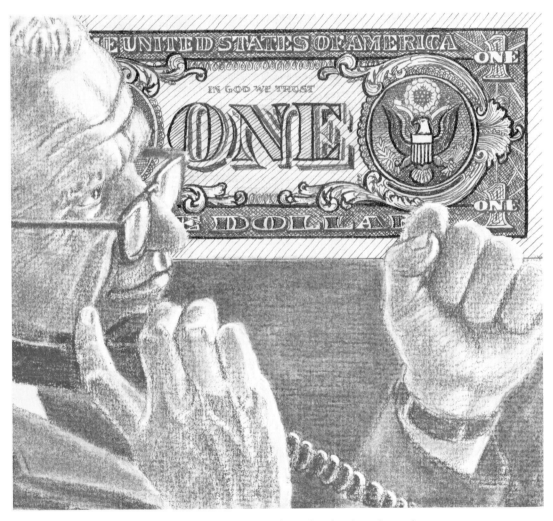

The negative aspect of desire is the obsession
to fill our emptiness with people and things.

of things that we have done in the past and we are angry at ourselves for doing those things. This kind of anger is positive anger at our negative self. It is good to feel guilty about that negativity, otherwise we would not experience our positivity and know the difference between right and wrong.

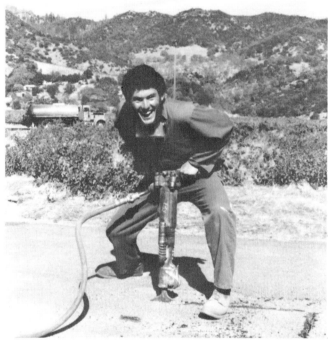

Warmth and power are two positive qualities of fire.

Anger creates movement and allows us to feel hungry, another by-product of the fire. That hunger, in its positive aspect, is feeling hunger for God. Each one of these emotions, when it is positive, is directed to the Lord. The problem with most therapies is that they teach us to focus our anger on someone else, like our mother or father, and let go of that anger toward ourselves. Actually, we need that anger so we can use its power to stop the negative things that we are doing in our lives and to actively choose more positive situations.

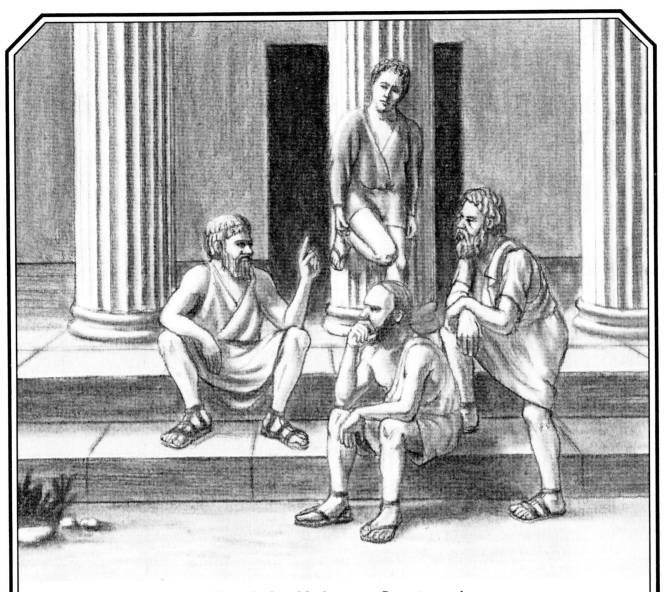

The relationship between Socrates and
his students illustrates positive attachment.

sciousness upward. Unfortunately, we are usually too full
of negative attachments to other people and things. We
have to switch that attachment, take the power of positive
attachment, and put it into the teacher.

Increasing our consciousness as we create actions in this
world will lead us to more positive attachments. The reactions that come back to us will be more positive because we
are conscious of how we create those reactions through our

own actions, actions which result from our attachments. Our vibration will increase and we will find better and better teachers, which is what we are all seeking. Finally, when we are ready, we will find "the teacher."

The search for a teacher is what motivates us to go to college, just as it motivates the lone Indian in the desert who is searching for the spiritual teacher to help him reach Nirvana. Both types of people are seekers. So we can use attachment, or love, in a positive way by seeking the Lord and attaching to Him.

Finally, fear is the fifth and last emotion produced in the ether through the combination of the dominant element of ether (space) with the earth element. The positive aspect of fear is fearing our negativity and our tendency to want to destroy ourselves. The positive aspect of fear in the world is our effort to keep the body alive; being conscious of whether we are going to drive off a cliff, burn our hand on a hot stove, or drown in water. The positivity is having a healthy fear for the purpose of maintaining this space suit we call our body.

Another positive aspect of fear is the fear of God. I do not mean the traditional idea that He is vengeful, but rather that we are aware of His omnipresence, that He is with us at all times and knows when we are acting against Him, against our soul, against our true self. With this awareness, we cannot be hypocrites and pray to the Lord for forgiveness for the negative things we consciously do in His presence. This positive fear is our built-in safety valve.

The negative aspect of fear is fearing the positive energy, fearing the good things that are coming to us to help lead us to the Lord. These can be things like being a vege-

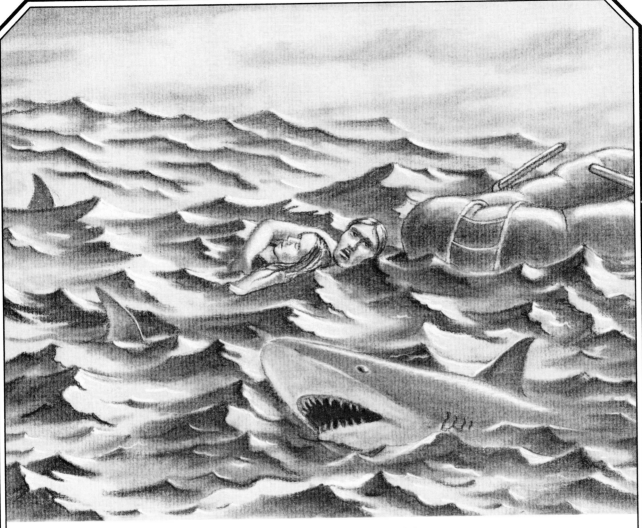

Courage is a positive aspect of fear.

tarian or doing emotional therapy work on ourselves in order to get to know who we are. The basest fear we have is the fear that we are not going to receive pleasure from all the things and relationships that we have in our lives.

By understanding the emotions, which are the physical stepdown of the five elements, we can begin to see how they affect the way in which we live our lives. We can learn to switch the negative aspects of all these emotions to their positive expressions. Then our lower self, our animal nature, will begin to reflect our soul quality.

Starting with the grossest emotion, the most crystallized energy of fear, we can learn to switch from the negative to the positive, from fear to courage, when we feel ourselves getting stuck. We can switch attachment to detachment, anger to warmth and compassion, desire to selflessness and humility, and grief to longing for the Lord.

When we have the courage to go through the pain, which means controlling the emotions, then we stop numbing ourselves. Going through the pain is very difficult because in the eyes of the world we are a fool if we are not numb to the pain in the world. If we are not taking drugs, drinking, sleeping around, and seeking pleasure, we are considered abnormal in this day and age.

The mind is habitual. It is stuck in the senses, in the material world. Human beings are creatures of habit. We just go around and around. We do things like the animals, over and over and over again. So when we start saying no to the senses, "No, I am not going to scatter my sexual energy anymore. No, I am not going to be angry. I am not going to put that food, that anger into my body. I am not going to scatter my mind and put it into indulgences and drugs," we stop being dead and numb and start being more alive and conscious.

We may look like fools in the eyes of the world because this new awareness has religious connotations. It means controlling our passions, the animal part of ourselves, our fear, our anger, and our desire. Most people do not like to control these passions. They want to explode them outwards. They want to indulge in these passions. They enjoy them.

For example, the mind says, "God, why haven't you given me a Rolls Royce?" Then the mind takes pleasure, an indulgence, in getting angry about what it does not have. Anger is a pleasure for most people, even though it is difficult for them to see it that way.

Instead of coming to the point of accepting life as it is dealt out to us, what do we do? We kill life. We kill the animals around us and take out our anger on them. Then what do we do? We eat the anger and wonder why we are so angry all the time. It is habitual. We slaughter in anger and eat the meat to have the pleasure and the taste. Then we wonder how we get more animal-like. It is because we have increased that energy of anger inside ourselves by constantly recycling it.

It takes courage to be "the fool" because our mind is tricky. Our mind forces us to indulge in the passions. Our mind squeezes our arm and pulls it behind our back and says, "Oh, having sex will feel so good. Oh, that meat will taste so good. Alcohol and cigarettes are so wonderful. What pleasure! Taste it, feel it, drink it, and smoke it. These pleasures will make you feel on top of the world." So we give in. We imbibe the drink, the smoke, the meat, the drugs, and the sexual experience without commitment. We absorb the pleasure, and we do not understand how we keep on getting the reaction of pain.

When we become conscious of our emotions, of our passions, we can accept them, all of them. We accept the fear, the attachment, the anger, the desire, and the grief. When we can accept our true grief, which is longing for God, then we can experience the nothingness. We can know that we are nothing. We have no-thing. When there is

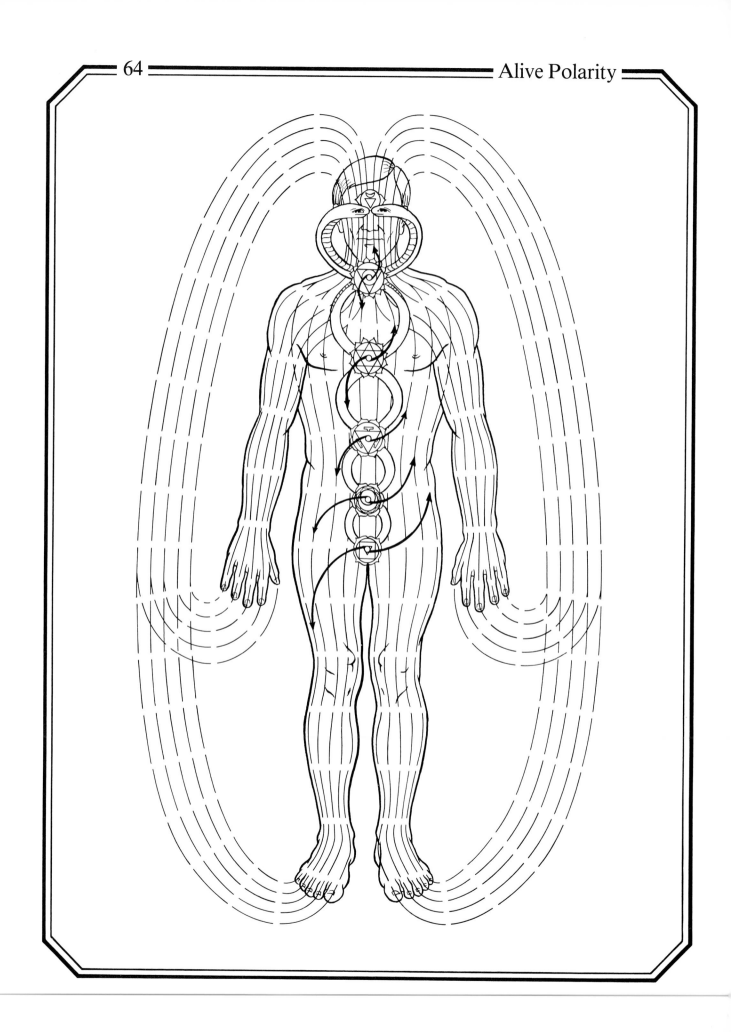

nothing, the past is gone; it has no relationship to us anymore. The future is not with us; it is coming. In between those two situations there is nothing. There is no-thing, so it becomes possible to have the acceptance of both the future and the past, which brings us into the now, the present.

When we are in the present, we have an understanding of where we are going. This relationship of the past, present, and future is another triangle, a reflection of the original triune function of the three principles of fire, air, and water. It is another stepdown of the three main energies that are the foundation of this universe.

Now we begin to see how the essence of mind creates the substance of form. The air principle, the Sattva, at the causal level, is the pathway for the soul to enter down the central core of the body. In the human body, the causal level occurs above the third eye in the upper regions of the mental realm. The fire principle, the Raja energy, and the water

The longitudinal electromagnetic waves (broken lines) flow over the entire surface of the body and through the muscular structure. These energy waves extend beyond the skin about one half inch, forming a protective energy envelope. The waves shown here are diagrammatic only and show the arrangement of the flow.

The snakes are part of the caduceus, the ancient Egyptian healing symbol of the major principles of energy in the body. The snakes are the energy, which is the true healer. Here they represent the energy currents as they generate a chakra or energy center at each crossover in the new body. The chakras step down the energy at each level to give power to the physical functions that each chakra governs.

Note the spin direction of each of the five lower chakras and how each chakra generates two lines of force: one motor current (outgoing) and one sensory current (returning).

principle, the Tamas energy, split from the air principle, the Sattva energy, at the eye center which is the sixth chakra, the astral level. From there, the energy weaves downward in a spiralling, serpentine movement to create the five lower chakras.

The Raja moves down to the right eye and out through the right ear, and the Tamas moves down to the left eye and out through the left ear. They cross over and meet at the throat, connecting once again with the air energy at the central core of the developing body. Here at the throat, the ether chakra is formed, the first and highest of the physical chakras in the body. Of the seven chakras in the body, the top two are in the spiritual and mental realms and the bottom five are physical.

At the throat, the ether chakra is created by a spinning motion of the three principles. These currents radiate upwards and downwards from the center of each chakra and spin outwards to weave the physical body. As the energy moves downward in the body, the vibration becomes one of denser and denser matter. Each succeeding chakra, from the ether, to the air, to the fire, water, and earth, is created by this same movement.

The particular emotions of grief, desire, anger, attachment, and fear form the physical vibration. Remember now that the original five elements have formed physically into five emotions within the ether, or fifth chakra, located at the throat. These emotions then combine and re-combine. The energy slows down as it gets further away from its Source, and the emotions become more and more crystallized. Combinations occur in each successively lower chakra as the dominant emotion of each chakra interacts

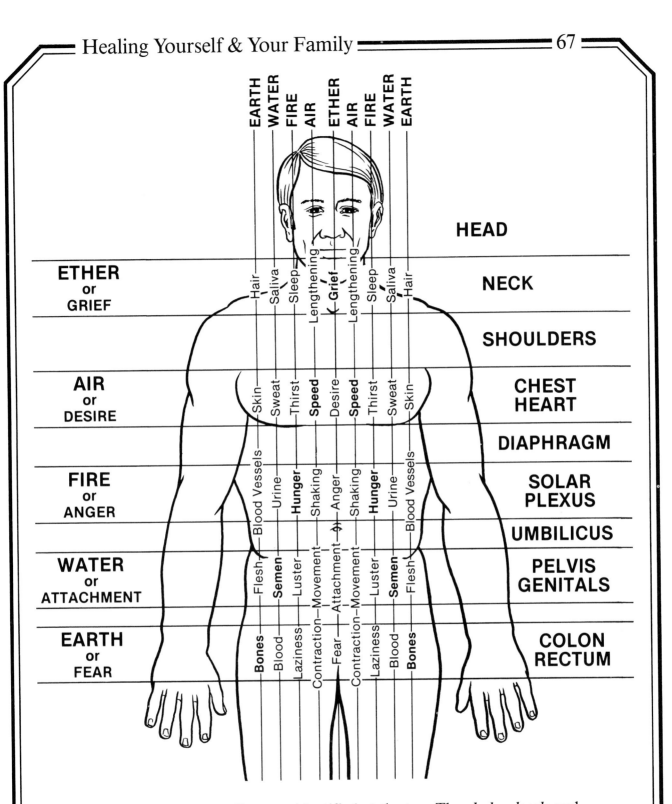

The *bi-polar current lines* are identified at the top. The *chakra levels* and their dominant emotions are shown on the left. Where the lines and the chakra levels cross, we have a resulting combination. These two factors are the "warp and woof" that weave the emotions and the physical body. The *main products* of each element are shown in bold type.

with the other four. This interaction is how the physical body is created.

For example, the emotions step down from the fifth chakra where the dominant emotion of the space is grief. This emotional energy slows down and crystallizes into the fourth chakra where the dominant emotional quality of the air is desire. This chakra is located in the center of the chest. It is here that we take in our first breath. We take oxygen (air or prana) into our body, which activates all the emotions, all the elements that were latent until that moment. In this fourth chakra we are dealing with the production of gases in the body.

The main physical quality of desire (air), before it interacts with any other emotions, is speed. We move out into the world and the world is made up of speed, and the speed is a physical manifestation of desire.

When desire (air), as the dominant emotion, combines with grief (ether), it produces lengthening; with anger (fire), it produces shaking; with attachment (water), it creates movement; and with fear (earth), it produces contraction. These qualities are all part of the physical make-up of the body. When we feel desire emotionally, the way it manifests physically in the body is through shaking, moving, contracting, or lengthening. When I see someone shaking, I know that they are going through desire as their main emotional block.

As the energy slows down a little more we find ourselves in the third chakra, located at the solar plexus. Here the dominant emotional quality of fire is anger. The main physical quality of anger (fire) is hunger. When the anger interacts with the other four emotions, we can see what the heat of the fire produces. When the dominant emotion of anger interacts with grief, we get sleep; with desire, we get thirst; with attachment, we have lustre or radiance; and with fear, we get laziness.

Continuing in the crystallization process we move into the fluids of the water chakra, the second chakra. Attachment, or love, is the dominant emotional quality in this chakra, which is located in the area of the generative organs of the body. Semen is the main physical quality of attachment. When the emotion of attachment becomes physical, it manifests as the fluid in the body which propagates the species. This fluid is semen in a man and the egg in a woman.

When attachment combines with the other four emotions in this second chakra, the other fluids of the body are produced. For example, when the dominant emotion of attachment mixes with grief, it creates saliva; with desire, it creates sweat; with anger, it produces urine; and with fear, it creates blood.

Finally, the vibrational effect is slowed down as far as it goes in the human body when the spinning energy creates the earth chakra, the first chakra, located at the base of the spine in the area of the bowels. This is where the solids are produced by the combination of the dominant emotion of fear, from the earth element, with the other four emotions. The main physical quality of fear (earth) is bones. When fear, the dominant emotion, interacts with grief, we get hair; with desire, we get skin; with anger, we get blood vessels; and with attachment, we get flesh.

These emotions, these particular vibrations of the elements, have a direct relationship with one another. When we go through any fear it will affect all the minerals we have in our body. If we have fear, we are immediately leaching the minerals that are in the bones. The dominant emotion of the earth is fear and the main quality of earth in the physical body is the bones. If there is a problem in the blood vessels we can bet it has to do with fear and anger. The physical emotions create the problem with the physical body. When we have a strong negative or unhealthy attachment, it is immediately going to affect the blood. When the attachment to our mother or father, our "blood," is out of balance, we create blood diseases like leukemia.

Physical disease occurs because of the crystallization of negative emotions in our bodies. The emotional energy begins at the top of the body in the ether, the fifth chakra. When that emotion of grief is healthy and positive, it goes toward the Lord. When it becomes negative, we initiate a downward spiral of dis-ease. Here is how a downward spiral can work. First we have longing, and instead of directing that longing toward God, we get obsessed and long for a mate. Then the energy drops down and we get desire. Instead of desiring the Lord, we find that we desire another person. When we do not get our desire fulfilled, we get angry at the other person because we are not getting what we want. When we get angry, we get attached to the negativity of the anger; we get attached to the other person. We get so locked into the other person, we drop downward once again and find ourselves afraid that they will be taken away from us. We have fear that they will leave us. This downward spiral is what creates the pain that we experience in our body and mind, which in turn creates disease.

The relationship between the body, mind, and emotions

is direct; each is inextricably bound to the other. This connection means that if something is going on in one area, we can be sure it is also happening at other levels. For example, if we are sick in the physical body, it means that we have already been sick and unbalanced at the emotional level for a long time. It takes a while for the more subtle emotional imbalances to crystallize down into the physical body.

When we work through our emotions, and accept our pain, we will then come to the point of accepting our physical body, because our body is our emotions. Our body is made up of reactions: the heart that is beating, the breaths we are taking, and the manner in which we are eliminating. After all, our body is a result of a reaction, the union of our parents, the explosion of the sperm and the egg. When we can come to the point of recognizing that our body is made up of reactions, we will realize and accept everything in us as reactionary. We will see that we live in a world of reaction, of duality, of polarity. There is no way we can escape this polarity while we live on this planet.

Once we accept ourselves as a bundle of reactions, we will begin to react less to other people. This equanimity is the key to life. Emotionally, we usually don't want to cop to our reactions. We know that, physically, when we get stuck by a thorn in the body, it is very painful. When we take that thorn out, it is not so painful anymore and we stop reacting. In the same way, as we become more conscious of our emotions and how our mind works, we will "remove the thorns" and we will begin to react less and less. Then someone can come up to us and yell at us and call us names, they can do whatever it is they do to test us, and pretty soon they will give up because we have stopped reacting.

People can say, "You're ugly," and we can say, "Thank you." They can say, "I hate you," and we can say, "I understand." Because we do understand. We are being real. In other words, we have learned agreement. We learn to agree. We can say, "Yes, I've been looking at that part of myself for about a year now and it's really bothering me. Can you help me please?" And since they have only looked at that part of us for a moment they say, "Help you, I don't even know you!"

So what I'm talking about is turning that negative reactionary energy into healing energy. We can call it emotional alchemy. It is transmuting the negative into the positive for our own healing.

IV

Alive Astrology:
How the Emotions Weave the Body

There is a form of science that has been heavily criticized over many years because it has not been understood by the scientific community, and that science is called astrology. I really did not understand astrology either until one day someone was telling me about it and said, "Jeff, astrology deals with gravity. It is about our relationship to that force. We usually do not pay much attention to gravity. We walk around this earth and we just expect to stand up."

Well, one day, back when I used to fish, I was thinking about this statement. I knew that the best time to fish was when there was a full moon. So I would always wait for a full moon to go fishing because that was when the fish would bite best. It was then I realized that the tides have a great effect on the fish, too. I started to see that if the moon can affect the fish and the pull of the water on the entire earth, then it must also affect my body, which I was told in my anatomy class was made up of about eighty percent water.

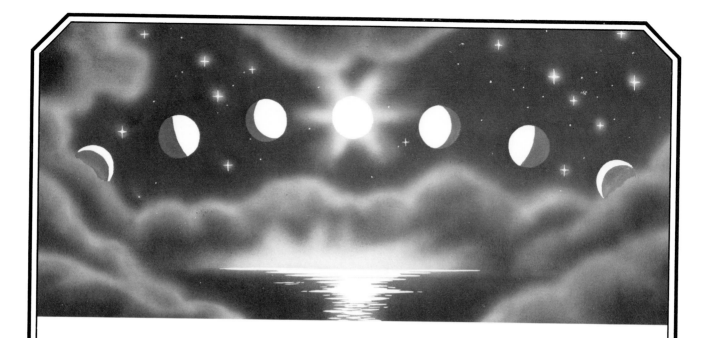

When I saw that the moon was affecting my body, moving me up and down, I saw how it definitely related to women and the menstrual cycles they go through. Women are more receptive to the moon than men. The moon never used to appeal to me and now it does. Now I recognize that there is a subtle force of gravity, a pull that tugs on our insides. That force pulls the water, which pulls the emotions, which then creates lovemaking, which then creates a physical body.

Finally I began to give some credence to astrology. I figured if the moon can do what I have described, then definitely other planets that are around this earth also have their effect. So I started to accept astrology. Then I met Dr. Randolph Stone who had a section on astrology in one of his books showing how the zodiac affects the weaving of the human body within the womb.

Dr. Stone taught me that out of the basic three principles comes the ether chakra of the new body that grows in the womb. Out of the ether comes the development of the next four chakras which create the physical matter that makes up the body. The ether develops the whole emotional foundation within the body-mind. The main emotional quality of the ether, which is our emotional reactionary base, relates to the feeling of grief about our predicament here on earth; that we really come out of nothing and at the same time we are attracted to everything. Out of that grief comes desire, and out of desire follows anger, attachment (love), and fear. These emotional forces start to weave and create the physical body, in which the soul will become trapped and thus dominated by the body-mind on this plane.

Astrology serves as a way to understand how the elemental energies, represented by the twelve signs of the zodiac, come down into matter and affect who we are. The weaving process of the body follows the signs of the zodiac in chronological order, with each sign governing the growth of some part of the body-mind. This weaving process helps us understand more fully how every sign of the zodiac is within each one of us.

The weaving starts at the head, which is the energy of Aries. Aries is the creative fire, the initiator, the leader, the starter. It is the ramming energy we see when a baby is born, as it rams its head against the mother in its effort to come into this world and out of the ether. The negative aspect of Aries is the "me first" energy. Aries, at the head, begins the cycle of the zodiac that ends in the feet, which are governed by Pisces.

So the Aries energy creates the head and the head is where the brain resides. The brain is the most subtle matter in our body. The brain is where the consciousness develops. It is also where the weaving activity begins its descent into the rest of the body.

As we move away from the head, we move down through the nervous system to the neck and the Taurus energy. The earth energy of Taurus is the neck. Emotionally, this is where we have our pride and our stubbornness. At the neck, our whole physical entity has moved from the Aries energy of the brain, the energy of pushing out into the world and the fire of creativity, down into the neck, to the earthly essence of Taurus.

Then the weaving continues from Taurus into the airy energy of Gemini. The Gemini energy in the shoulders has to do with the physical aspect of the world, carrying the world on our shoulders. When we have stuffed and stored our worldly worries, our shoulders are pushed downward and inward. The brachial plexus between the shoulders controls the diaphragm and the chest. The shoulders either constrict that area or expand it. When the shoulders relax, the whole breathing process can take place naturally. Asthma, for instance, is a Gemini block because the emotion of desire (from the air) constricts the brachial plexus, which then constricts the chest.

Next, the energy moves and weaves downward from the air energy of the shoulders to the water energy of Cancer, in the breast and heart. The energy of the breast and heart is our relationship to our home. Everything that is centered around our heart is our home. When our heart and our rhythm stop, we lose our home which is the body.

Cancer, the crab, has a shell. During the weaving process, the soul is moving into its shell just like a crab. Cancers are always looking for better shells to live in. We human beings are always looking for a better body to live in

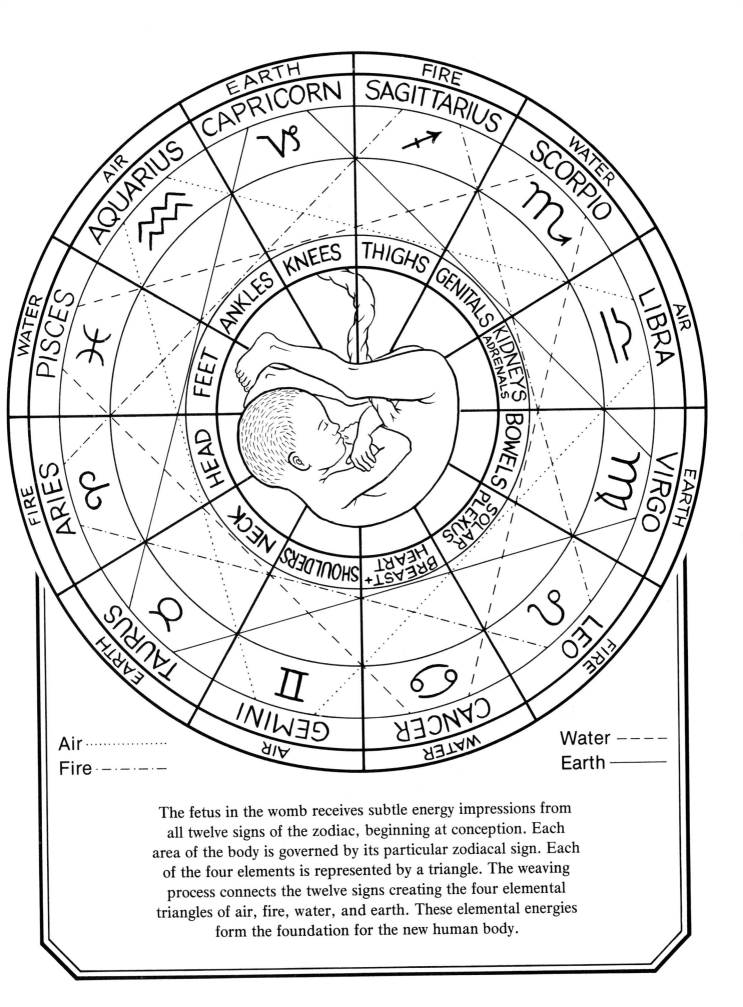

EARTH CAPRICORN ♑ · FIRE SAGITTARIUS ↗ · WATER SCORPIO ♏ · AIR LIBRA ♎ · EARTH VIRGO ♍ · FIRE LEO ♌ · WATER CANCER ♋ · AIR GEMINI ♊ · EARTH TAURUS ♉ · FIRE ARIES ♈ · WATER PISCES ♓ · AIR AQUARIUS ♒

KNEES · THIGHS · GENITALS · KIDNEYS · ADRENALS · BOWELS · SOLAR PLEXUS · BREAST + HEART · SHOULDERS NECK · HEAD · FEET · ANKLES

Air ·············
Fire —·—·—·—

Water — — — —
Earth ——————

The fetus in the womb receives subtle energy impressions from all twelve signs of the zodiac, beginning at conception. Each area of the body is governed by its particular zodiacal sign. Each of the four elements is represented by a triangle. The weaving process connects the twelve signs creating the four elemental triangles of air, fire, water, and earth. These elemental energies form the foundation for the new human body.

because we usually do not like the one we have.

The positive aspect of the Cancer energy is that it makes the body, our form, strong. It strengthens our acceptance of our physical limitations. It creates a strong protection so the body-mind does not get destroyed by negativity. The Cancer energy teaches us that we can have a positive form and live peacefully within it, within ourselves. We can protect ourselves from negativity and at the same time be part of that negativity, because there has to be a certain degree of negativity in order for us to exist. The polarity of negativity and positivity is the nature of matter on this physical plane.

The next development, as our energy descends and becomes more dense and crystallized, is the fire of Leo. Inside our body, the fire is centered at the solar plexus which is created by the Leo energy during the weaving process. The solar plexus is the place from which the fire energy radiates creativity outward. It is the radiant sun that we see in the sky. We are able to receive the sun's energy through our solar plexus, inside ourselves, and give out that fire to others through the warmth that flows from our eyes. We are able to receive that blessing of radiant energy and incorporate it into the human form, the human body. We do that through the solar plexus.

At the solar plexus, one of two things can happen: we can expand our energy and get it moving upward, towards the diaphragm and back to where we came from at birth, back to God; or we can constrict the life force, the fiery energy of creativity, and move downward. When we constrict that flame and attempt to smother it, the energy moves downward, and we become more emotional and more unconscious. We create more and more pleasures in our lives which, in our world of duality, of polarity, necessarily bring us more and more pain.

The spiralling energy continues to weave the new body inside the womb. It leaves the solar plexus and moves into the earth energy of Virgo, which is our bowels, where we absorb our food. The Virgo energy is very much one of nurturing and one of service. It knows how to receive and utilize the nurturing energy of food, in physical terms from the bowels, as well as how to exchange nurturing energy with others. Almost all Virgos I have ever known have had something to do with service and have given lots of attention to their bowels.

The next energy that is developed is the Libran air, which is the kidneys and the adrenals. This energy determines the balance within a person. The kidneys govern energy as it moves throughout the body. The development of the adrenals, which produce adrenalin, allows us to stay in balance with the sensitivity that we have so the energy can flow freely through us. The kidneys govern the balance between the body, mind, and spirit.

The weaving continues downward to the water energy of Scorpio, which is the generative energy in the body. Here in the pelvis lies the focus of our emotional life. Within the pelvis, the water basin, we have the generative organs which create new life. Scorpio energy here in the pelvis is like a dam that has been created in the body. The dam is built up to give force to our emotions so they move through us and outwards to other people. The sexual energy of Scorpio enables us to reproduce ourselves through emotional attraction.

In the womb, the fetal position of the child looks like a squat. The only difference from the squat is that the feet are pulled inward and upward. The hands are folded to each side and the arms are wrapped around the body and the legs. It is in this position that the fire of Sagittarius creates the thighs as the descending energy continues to crystallize. The Sagittarian energy is the movement of the body. It allows the movement of the child within the womb in the same way the thighs allow the movement of the body when we walk out in the world.

The Sagittarian energy of fire is the one that is able to explore and see everything that is around it. Sagittarian energy is what creates more understanding of what is around us. Then, once we see the truth of something, we start to have ideals. The positive force of the Sagittarian energy is that the ideals it creates can move us upwards towards oneness in the world. The negative aspect of the fire of Sagittarius is that its power can also move us downwards where we end up forcing ourselves into more and more negativity. We become so blurred in our vision that we are unable to see what is ahead of us.

Moving down, the next energy developed is at the knees, the Capricorn energy. Capricorn is an earth energy. It is one of stability and firmness. It is one that creates power through stability and self-assurance. Capricorn energy teaches that we can only find stability as long as we surrender, go down on our knees and kneel to the One energy, to the Lord. The Capricorn energy, when it is positive, recognizes that being stable and confident comes only through humility, when we are surrendering to something greater than ourselves. The Capricorn energy of the knees teaches us about the power of kneeling in surrender while we are in this world, as well as the recognition that there is something more than just this world of physical matter.

The next energy is the air of Aquarius, in the ankles. Aquarius is the energy that allows the fish of Pisces to swim underwater and to breathe at the same time. The Aquarian energy enables us to have the understanding of truth and give it to others. It is the energy that creates the ankles, which allow human beings to stand up and walk into this world on their own two feet and understand what truth and honesty are all about. The Aquarian energy is visionary. It has the quality of seeing what the future can bear.

The final weaving in the womb is that of the feet, which embody the water energy of Pisces. The Pisces energy is the last part of the water principle: the bi-polar energy current that moves from head to foot, up and down, and creates the physical form of the body.

The feet are the negative pole of the brain. We can see the physical manifestation of our chronic mind patterns when we look at the configuration of our feet. When we do not deal with negative mental and emotional energy it becomes crystallized in our bodies. Gravity pushes that energy downwards and eventually the negative energy gets stuck in the feet. We feel that blockage in our feet as pain. In the feet is the accumulation of chronic karma from our past lives and emotional and mental pain from our present life.

We can learn to read the feet by understanding how the five toes are the five emotions made visible. Each toe represents one of the five elements of ether, air, fire, water, and earth. Each toe corresponds to the triune function of each of the elements, as represented by the signs of the zodiac. For example, the earth toe is the earth chakra which is made up of the Taurus, Capricorn, and Virgo energies. Since the zodiacal energies weave the different parts of the physical body, the earth toe can then be read as containing the reflex points to the neck, knees, and bowels. Emotionally, the earth toe corresponds to the positive and negative attributes of each of the earth signs. The positive aspect of Taurus is humility; Virgo, service; and Capricorn, surrender. We will be able to see the emotional work that needs to be done to enhance our positivity by reading our toes.

One of the ways we can read the toes is by checking for distortions in their arrangement on the feet. For example, if our earth toe is extremely small and curled underneath the water toe, we know we are holding a great deal of negativity in our mind and emotions in the form of fear.

General map of the regional energy relationships. The feet, as a whole, have an energy reflex to the pelvis and neck. Also, specific parts of the feet have specific reflexes: for example, the transverse arch of the foot affects the diaphragm, and the ball of the foot affects the chest. Pains in specific parts of the feet reflect an impeded energy flow in the corresponding reflex points and vice versa. Proper manipulation of these areas will re-establish the flow.

Positive, negative, and neuter poles have a definite energy relationship. Any influence that has an effect on one pole will affect the other two, demonstrating the Hermetic Principle, "As above, so below."

Also, note that working on the large toe and inside edge of the foot affects the energy flow on the ether line and the ether chakra. Work on the earth toe and the outside edge of the foot affects the earth line and the earth chakra and all its corresponding functions in the body, and so on.

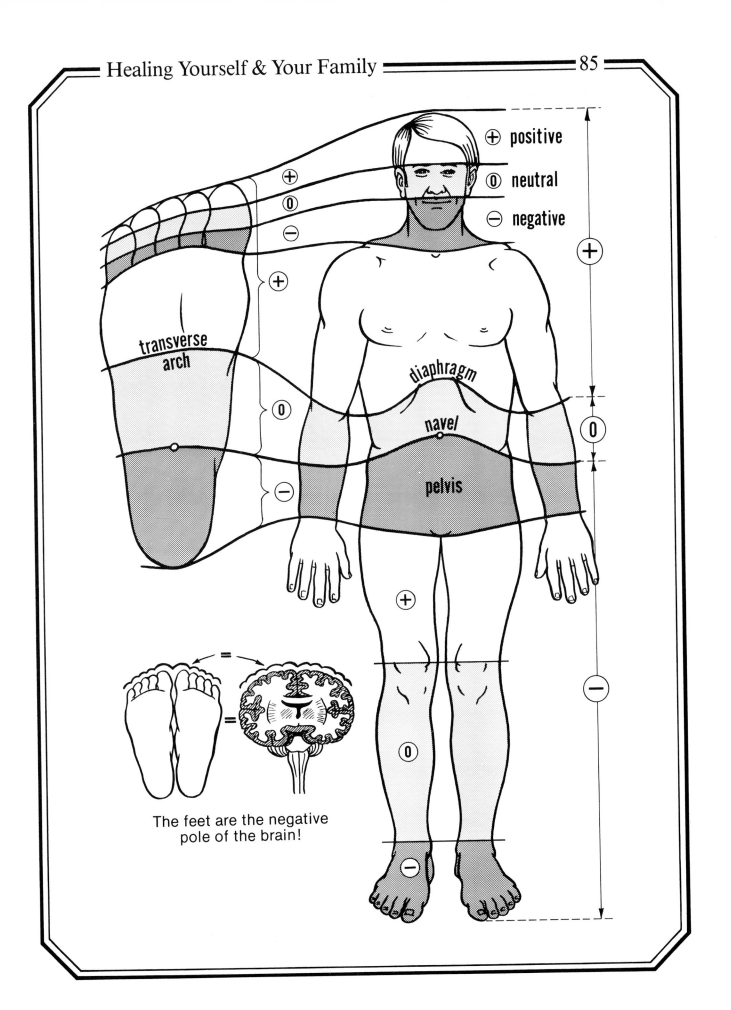

⊕ positive

⓪ neutral

⊖ negative

transverse arch

diaphragm

navel

pelvis

The feet are the negative pole of the brain!

Reading the feet according to Alive Astrology

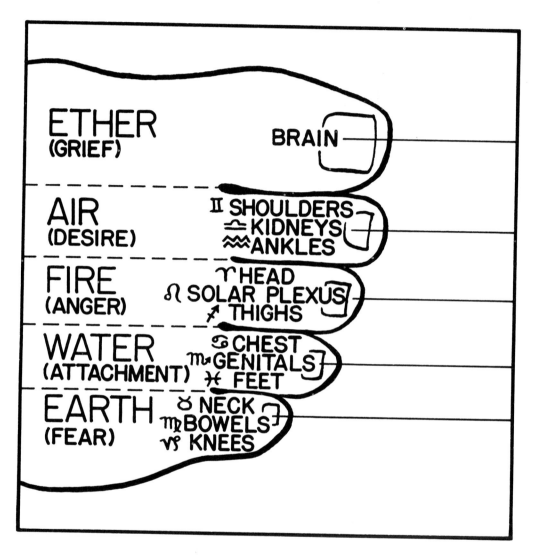

ETHER
(GRIEF)

BRAIN

AIR
(DESIRE)

♊ SHOULDERS
♎ KIDNEYS
♒ ANKLES

FIRE
(ANGER)

♈ HEAD
♌ SOLAR PLEXUS
♐ THIGHS

WATER
(ATTACHMENT)

♋ CHEST
♏ GENITALS
♓ FEET

EARTH
(FEAR)

♉ NECK
♍ BOWELS
♑ KNEES

This foot shows normal toes with the bi-polar current
lines labelled: ether, air, fire, water, earth. Each toe,
as a whole, incorporates the physical reflexes governed by
each astrological sign. Working on a specific toe affects
all three physical areas, as well as the corresponding emotion.

Example of chronic fear

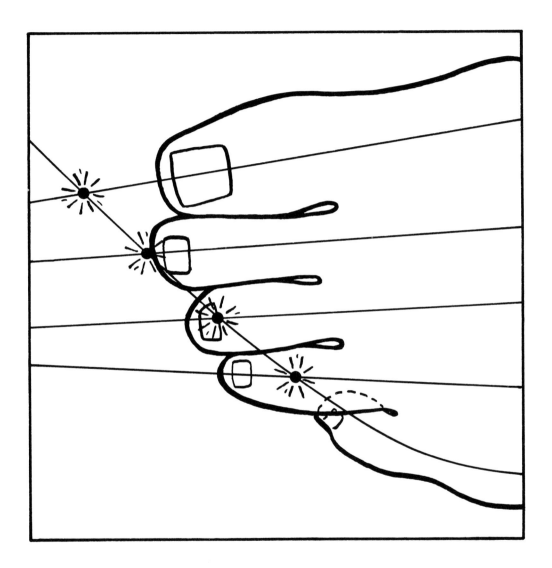

This foot, drawn from a live subject, shows energy
lines traced through the axis of each toe. Notice how the
emotion of fear crosses over and "short circuits" the
corresponding energy lines of the other toes, showing how
chronic fear drains energy from the other chakras.

Once we recognize the weakness, we can switch our emotional negativity to positivity by exaggerating and encouraging the positive attributes of each of the three zodiacal signs that are contained within each toe. Specifically, with the earth toe, we can work emotionally on the humility of Taurus, the surrender of Capricorn, and the service of Virgo. Physically, we may be prone to constriction and blockage in our neck, knees, and bowels. Since we know that the elements are the emotions and the emotions are what actually create the physical body, we can see in the toes exactly where our work lies.

Actually, in reflexology, the entire foot can be mapped to correspond to every part of the body. When we understand and accept that each part of the foot is a reflex point to another part of the body, we will be able to read the feet as we would a life history. We will be able to identify all our chronic negative mind patterns on a physical and emotional level.

The Piscean energy at the feet completes us in our effort to become grounded in this world and at the same time helps us to understand the relationship of the earth to God. The Piscean energy teaches us that the earth and everything on it came out of the water after the One energy split into

The horizontal bands (dotted lines) show the relationship of the back of the feet to the spine and the internal organs. Specific reflex points have been omitted deliberately to encourage individual awareness in relating the sore spots on the back of the feet to the sore spots on the back. Energy flow can be facilitated by the use of two hands: one on each corresponding sore spot, above and below. When done properly, this has a powerful polarizing and balancing effect on the related energy fields.

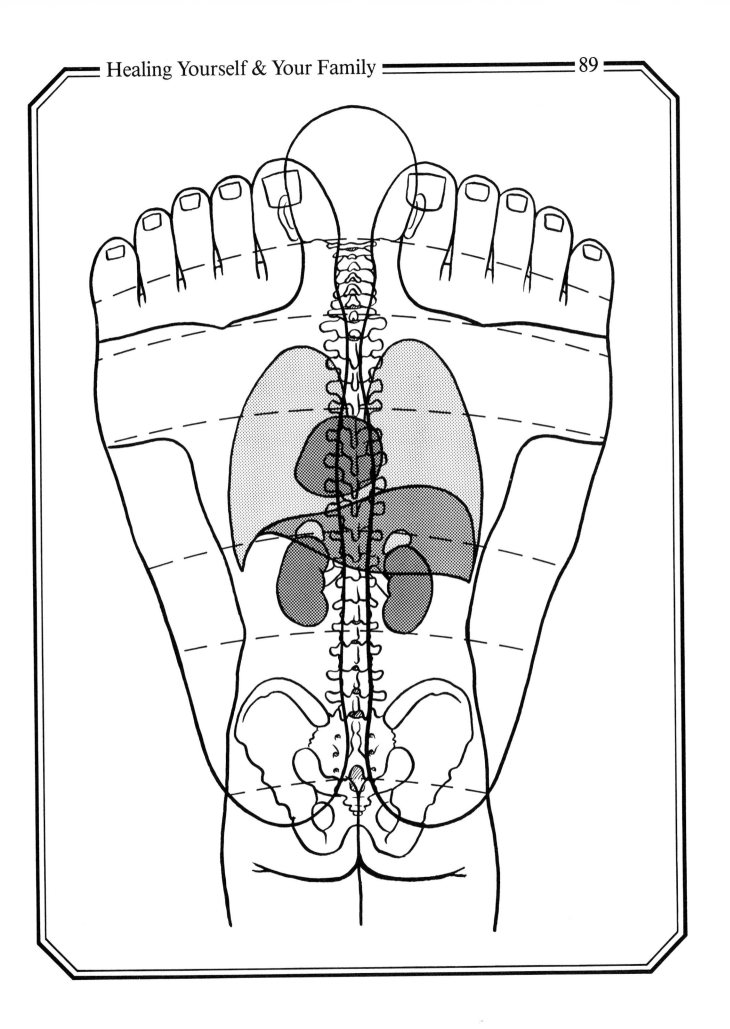

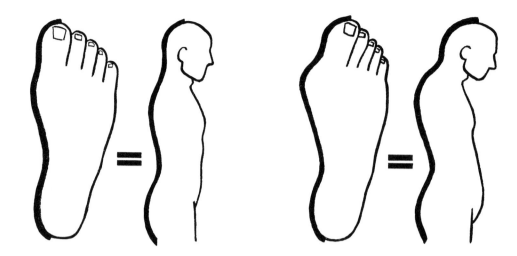

Imbalances indicated in the feet foretell eventual changes in the structure and function of related parts of the body.

three. Through this understanding, we can see how the spiritual essence is all around us on this earthly plane. The key for Pisceans is to become grounded so they know and love the earth, which will then bring them to know and love the spirit. All this understanding comes because Pisces is the furthest away from the head but the closest to the spirit. Once we are far enough away from the Source, then we can recognize the Source. Separation creates longing for the One. When we are close to the Source, we do not experience that longing. We cannot see the Source until we step back. Then we can see.

When the Piscean energy has made its contribution, the weaving process of the entire body is complete inside the womb. Each sign of the zodiac represents a specific element which corresponds to a specific emotion. This emotional energy that weaves the body has stepped down from the forces of the outer energies, from the planets as they rule the signs of the zodiac, and has created our fingers and our toes: the physical manifestation of the five different elements in the body.

The first element is the ether, which is where the emotional development begins in the body. Then, out of this ether, from which all the physical is created, comes the air. The air element is made up of the three air signs of Gemini, Aquarius, and Libra. Those three energies create another triune function within the body, a stepdown of the original trinity of the three principles of fire, air, and water. The original trinity of principles that stepped down from the soul to the mind is now being repeated by each element in the physical body.

The next triune function is of fire. The fire trinity is composed of Aries, Leo, and Sagittarius. The third trinity we have in our body is the water element, which is made up of the Cancer, Scorpio, and Piscean energies. The densest trinity is the earth element: Taurus, Virgo, and Capricorn. So the original three principles, the triune function from the mind's blueprint, have stepped down through the ideas of the elements, to the action of the emotions, to the reaction of the physical body. This stepdown process creates another triune function made up of the causal, astral, and physical regions, the three levels through which the soul's energy travels in its descent.

The elemental energies that are being developed in the ether do not become active until the child takes its first breath. These energies are latent or inactive until the airy principle, the prana from the mind region, steps down. Then the soul, the child, comes into the world from the ether and actually breathes. Then the five elements attract

TRIUNE FUNCTION OF EACH ELEMENT

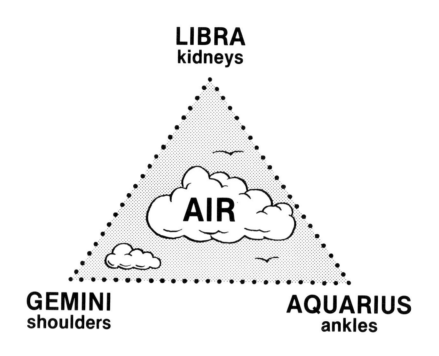

LIBRA
kidneys

AIR

GEMINI
shoulders

AQUARIUS
ankles

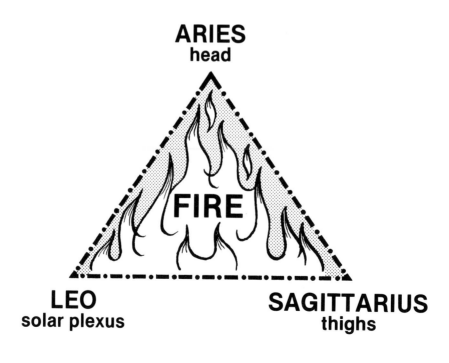

ARIES
head

FIRE

LEO
solar plexus

SAGITTARIUS
thighs

These four elemental triangles have been lifted out of the zodiac chart to show more clearly how the zodiacal signs are arranged according to their elements.

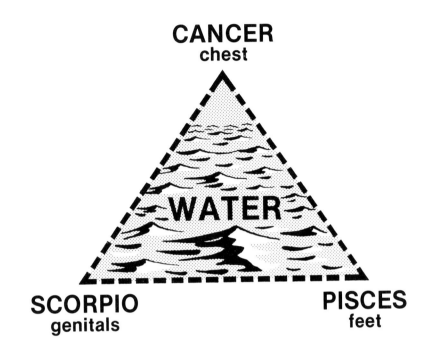

CANCER
chest

WATER

SCORPIO
genitals

PISCES
feet

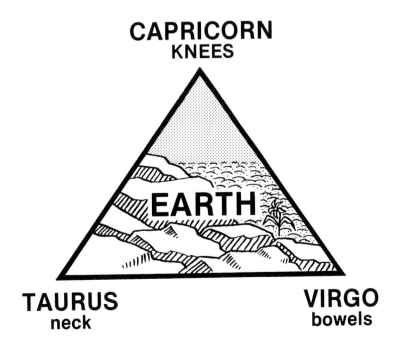

CAPRICORN
KNEES

EARTH

TAURUS
neck

VIRGO
bowels

their like elements from the outer forces of the planets. These elements are drawn to each other by the homeopathic principle of "like attracts like."

The moment of our first breath fixes our astrological chart. The outer forces of the planets and their position in the heavens make the imprint of how our inner patterns will be manifested through our actions in the world. Our astrological chart shows the potential of how our past actions, our original blueprint, can become our present and future, depending upon the work we do on ourselves. When we choose to do so, we can switch the negativity of our past to consciousness in the present and positivity in the future.

The newborn child is able to identify with the emotions of the father and mother because the parents' emotions are the original energy that started the development of the child's physical body. It is their emotional attraction to one another that draws them together to have sex. It is their emotions that the child absorbs and incorporates into its inner patterns while it grows in the womb.

For this reason, it is so important that our consciousness be very high and that we feel very good about ourselves as parents when there is a child in the mother's womb. The growing child is going to work on us; it is going to force out our negative emotions. If we suck them right up again, stuff them back inside ourselves, the child will absorb them until the emotions finally become crystallized. Then they will get stuck in the body of the child and the parents will have to deal with that negative energy for the rest of their lives. We cannot escape from our own karma. This fact becomes very clear when we have our own children. Our children are us and we are our children. As householders, God gives us an opportunity to do our work, parents and children alike.

Our work is mapped out for us in the triangle of our three main astrological signs: our sun, moon, and rising sign. The way I often work with people, physically and emotionally, is by looking at their three main elemental signs. This triangle creates the original foundation for each person at their birth. It deals with the principles and the elements within each individual's make-up.

I look at the sun sign as the way the soul manifests, the moon sign as the emotions, and the rising sign as the filter. The sun is the primary energy of the person and reflects what the father was going through at the time of conception. The moon is the secondary energy, the feminine energy of the mother at the time of conception. The moon energy reflects the sun. It is romantic, sensitive, and very cooling. It is the energy of feeling very hot, jumping into a river or pond, and feeling the refreshing quality of that coolness. The rising sign is our mask, our personality and our body. It is formed by the attachment between us and our parents.

So, we can look at our lives and at the qualities of our three main signs and see the emotions our parents were going through at the time of our conception. We can see their work. This study is a beautiful way to start looking at ourselves and our parents. We can see their mistakes as well as the healing they were going through at the time. We can either be positive or negative with these energies. It is up to us to choose.

I'll use myself as an example. My sun sign is the fire sign

of Sagittarius. Physically, this has to do with my thighs. I have big thighs. Sagittarius has to do with quickness and with energy moving downward and outward into the world and then scattering. It is speedy, very speedy. Sagittarians make particularly good leaders, lawyers, philosophers, and judges. They have good discrimination when their energy is moving upward. When their energy is moving downward, Sagittarians make great alcoholics, drug addicts, and gamblers. So Sagittarius is my sun energy which moves outward. It is the creative, radiant part of myself. It is my primary energy.

My secondary energy, my moon sign, is fire from Leo. Physically, this is the solar plexus. I have a lot of solar plexus energy, as we can tell by my big belly. It is interesting that as soon as the Fellowship was created, my diaphragm just opened up and my stomach came out. I have an incredible amount of solar plexus power which is my moon, my emotions. I know how to work with the emotions.

There are two kinds of energy for each sign of the zodiac: male and female. For example, for men, the male Leo manifests. The male lion is the king. Emotionally, he is the authority of the jungle. The presence alone, of the male lion, is enough. He is confident and relaxed. He lies back and enjoys protecting his family through the strength of his own presence. He is a protector. In the Fellowship, I am the protector through the guidelines I have set up. That quality is my male Leo energy. So if anything comes along to attack the family, my male Leo lion suddenly roars and springs into action, taking care of it immediately. That protective energy describes my emotions. That energy is my solar plexus, my emotional self as a male Leo.

The female Leo is very different. The female lion is the hunter. The female goes out and gets the food for the kids and is constantly active. She moves all over the place. You do not know where she is going to be next. She is feared because of her skill in killing. That killer power is what creates fear of the female Leo energy.

So, I have described my sun and my moon. Now in order to know my primary and secondary energies (my soul and my emotions), we need to go through my filter which is my body and image. To find out about my creative and my receptive sides, we must move through my image which is my body.

My body is not really here. The body is an image we get caught up in. It is not us. If we can take a picture of something, that means it is physical and not real. It is that simple. So our image is our filter. The body is the filter of my two main energies, the masculine and the feminine, the sun and the moon.

I need to clean my filter, my rising sign, in order to manifest the positive attributes of my primary and secondary energies, my sun and my moon. For me to truly realize Sagittarian idealism and Leo's kindness, I need to be fair, which is the positive aspect of my Libra rising.

My body, my rising sign, is Libran air. Libra is balance. Physically, Libra relates to the kidneys. So my image is fairness and balance. You can receive me as long as you see the fairness and balance in my life. If you reject balance, then you will not understand me. You will not feel my energy. If you accept the balance I put out, you will be able to receive the kindness and protective quality of my Leo and the idealism of my Sagittarian overview.

Positive attributes of the elements as reflected in the Zodiacal signs

AIR

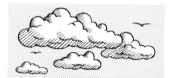

♊	Gemini	— Clarity
♒	Aquarius	— Honesty
♎	Libra	— Fairness

FIRE

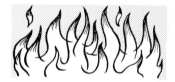

♈	Aries	— Responsibility
♌	Leo	— Kindness
♐	Sagittarius	— Idealism

WATER

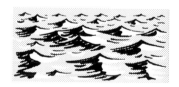

♏	Scorpio	— Receptivity
♓	Pisces	— Understanding
♋	Cancer	— Giving

EARTH

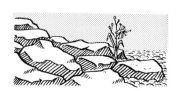

♑	Capricorn	— Surrender
♍	Virgo	— Service
♉	Taurus	— Humility

Attributes of our Three Main Astrological Signs

RISING
(neutral)
Physical body, personality, mask, energy filter

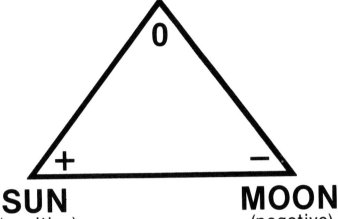

SUN
(positive)
Soul, male, outgoing
energy, mental body

MOON
(negative)
Emotions, female,
reflective energy, astral
or emotional body

Author's Three Main Astrological Signs

LIBRA
Fairness

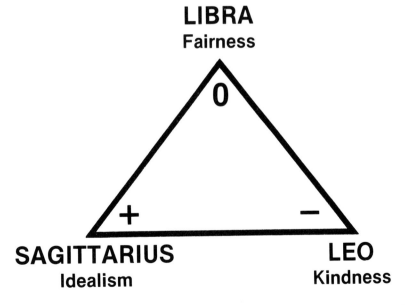

SAGITTARIUS
Idealism

LEO
Kindness

See positive attribute chart for your own personal
signs and apply them to your sun, moon, and
rising signs to discover your individual work.

In my body, the areas in which I show my energy are my thighs, my solar plexus, and my kidneys. On a physical level, my work definitely has been with my kidneys. They are getting better now. I am not retaining as much water as I used to. I tend to retain water, which is my emotions and other people's emotions, in my Libran body.

I am also very expansive, as you can tell from my solar plexus. I radiate warmth from my soul, my inner sun, my solar plexus, out to other people. You can get that warmth through the light in my eyes and the healing energy in my hands. It's funny how energy works. I picked a wife who is cool. We make a good combination. I warm her up and she cools me down.

So, what I have shared is my understanding of the correlation between the principles and the elements. I have shared about the Life: how it has moved from the energy of Oneness through to the mind. I have shown how that energy has stepped down to become the three principles of fire, air, and water. I have shared how these principles have stepped down to become the five elements, moving from the mind to the emotions within the womb at the time of conception, and there developing into the physical body.

When the body then steps out into the world, the prana, or life-breath, activates the five elements that were latent in the womb. The new human being begins its quest to understand where it has come from and where it is going, to understand life and death. From the moment a human being enters the world the pain begins. By going through the pain, each individual starts to learn his or her lessons for that lifetime.

In this world of polarity, we prefer pleasure and think

we will not have to experience pain. Pleasure is what numbs the mind. The mind is a callus that covers the soul. The mind does not want us to feel our pain. The mind wants us to forget our pain so that it can stay dominant and keep the soul trapped. Real freedom lies in remembering our pain and all the negative things we have done in our lives so that we never do them again.

True balance comes by recognizing our pain, becoming aware of our pain, and accepting it. Then we can forgive ourselves for the mistakes we have made. Only when we forgive ourselves are we able to forgive others. These times of higher consciousness in our lives are the life-death moments, the opportunities for major transition and change. These times are actually the real moments of birth because birth literally means "bringing to light."

Through understanding our pain, we can become more conscious and start to learn what the world is all about. We start to learn from the mistakes that have been created in this world. By learning from those mistakes, we grow and recognize the truth of what it means to take a human birth. We recognize that our body-mind is the temple of the Lord and that we have God inside ourselves. We gain the consciousness to move away from our emotional reactions and return to the Father. In this human birth we have the opportunity to learn about the Father (the Creative) and how His energy manifests from heaven to earth.

V

How to Live Happily by Healing Our Emotions

When we can accept the reactions in our lives, we will be able to accept the physical body and its imperfections. When we can accept the heaven and the hell that is in our bodies, the beauty and the ugliness, then we can accept the polarities. Then the mind reverses. The mind totally reverses and starts to give us the blueprint. We become less and less reactionary and more and more conscious. We gain understanding of how the mind works and rules us. Then we can use our consciousness to see how our present actions are a direct result of our past actions (both of pleasure and of pain) and how our present actions create our future. With this awareness we can learn to become more conscious of everything we do.

Awareness is learning to focus on our pain. It is learning the origin of our pain. Awareness is having the courage to go through that pain and become a more conscious human being in the process. The great people in history, the people who have helped humanity, are the people who have gone through their pain. Many have had some major trauma in their lives. They focused on that painful situation, gained the courage, and broke through to the other side. They switched their negativity to positivity. That ability is what creates geniuses and great humanitarians. What I want to impress upon everyone is that we all have that potential, that possibility; the qualities of being a genius and a great humanitarian are in each and every one of us.

Through awareness we start to recognize that pain is something from which we can learn. We can also learn from our pleasure, as well, because in this world of polarity we cannot have pleasure without pain. We cannot experience one side without a swing to the other side. If we get either a great deal of pain or a lot of pleasure, it is an opportunity to move through whatever that situation brings our way. In other words, when we have pain, we need to accept the pain. We must really focus on it and learn where the resistance lies. Then we can go through that resistance to the other side and experience the joy, the light, the understanding, and the new level of consciousness which that awareness brings.

When we focus on the pain that exists in our attachments to our parents, we start to become free of those attachments. We start to accept the mistakes our parents made and see that those mistakes are the same ones we made. Their mistakes are our mistakes because we are a combination of both our parents. Then an amazing thing happens. Instead of telling our parents what they should do, we start accepting what they have done. We start learning from our father being an alcoholic and accept his alcoholism so that we do not have to become an alcoholic ourselves. We see what ruled him and what brought him to that downfall. We accept his pain and recognize that his pain is our pain.

Then we understand that all the reaction we go through, from the physical pain in our bodies to the emotional and mental pain we experience, is happening to teach us certain things. That pain is there to bring us into greater and greater consciousness. And consciousness is acceptance. As we accept the reactions that are in this world, as we accept the war and the peace that are in this world, as we accept both sides of everything, then we can start to learn the main quality of what it is to be a human being, which is discrimination. We start to become discriminating. We know what is positive and conscious and what is negative and emotional.

The main quality of being human is having discrimination. Discrimination means knowing the difference between a destructive situation and a healing situation. As we start to go over the mistakes we have made in our lives, we begin to learn from them. We can even start to learn from the mistakes that have been made by others around us. We stop wanting to change the other person. Instead, we learn from their mistakes. We change. That is important. Most of the time we go around saying to others, "You should learn this and you should learn that," and so on. When we start taking responsibility for ourselves and our own lives, then we are the ones who do the changing.

We can actually learn from other people's mistakes, and that is great. We do not have to make the same mis-

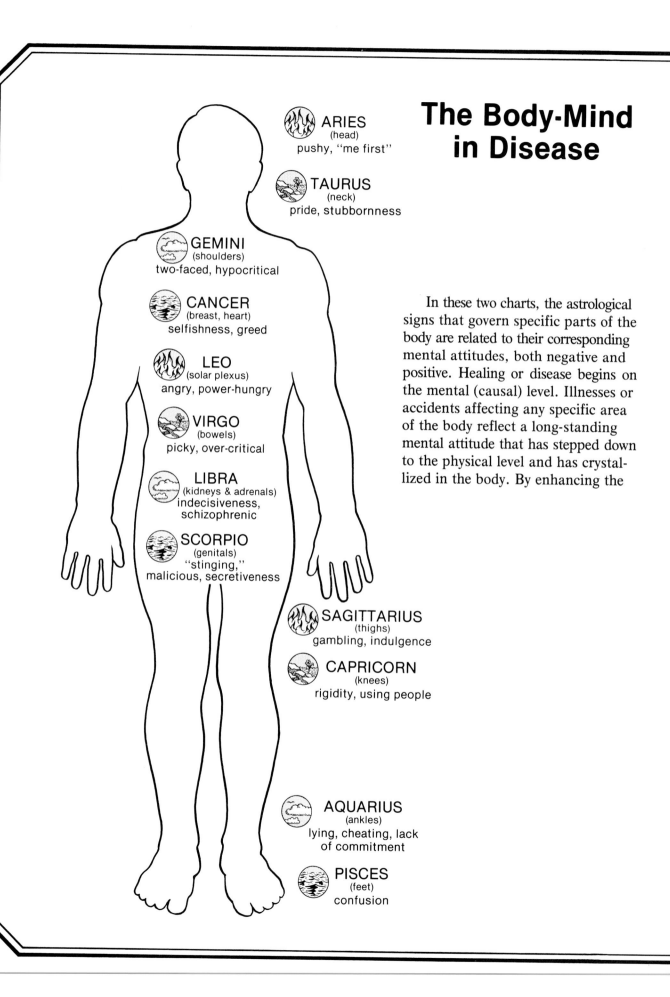

The Body-Mind in Disease

ARIES
(head)
pushy, "me first"

TAURUS
(neck)
pride, stubbornness

GEMINI
(shoulders)
two-faced, hypocritical

CANCER
(breast, heart)
selfishness, greed

LEO
(solar plexus)
angry, power-hungry

VIRGO
(bowels)
picky, over-critical

LIBRA
(kidneys & adrenals)
indecisiveness,
schizophrenic

SCORPIO
(genitals)
"stinging,"
malicious, secretiveness

SAGITTARIUS
(thighs)
gambling, indulgence

CAPRICORN
(knees)
rigidity, using people

AQUARIUS
(ankles)
lying, cheating, lack
of commitment

PISCES
(feet)
confusion

In these two charts, the astrological signs that govern specific parts of the body are related to their corresponding mental attitudes, both negative and positive. Healing or disease begins on the mental (causal) level. Illnesses or accidents affecting any specific area of the body reflect a long-standing mental attitude that has stepped down to the physical level and has crystallized in the body. By enhancing the

The Body-Mind in Healing

positive mental attitude which corresponds to the affected area of the body, we can assist the healing process. Likewise, since the flow of energy in the physical body affects the state of mind, energy balancing work which affects the specific areas of the body will help a person to switch from an old, negative and diseased mental attitude, to a new, positive, healing one.

ARIES
(head)
responsibility

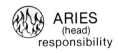
TAURUS
(neck)
constructive, persistent

GEMINI
(shoulders)
Clarity

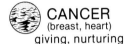
CANCER
(breast, heart)
giving, nurturing

LEO
(solar plexus)
kindness, warmth

VIRGO
(bowels)
serving, helpful

LIBRA
(kidneys & adrenals)
fairness, balance

SCORPIO
(genitals)
receptivity, regeneration

SAGITTARIUS
(thighs)
living our ideals
good judgment
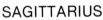

CAPRICORN
(knees)
surrender, prayerfulness
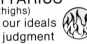

AQUARIUS
(ankles)
sincerity, honesty

PISCES
(feet)
understanding

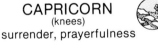

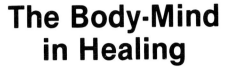

takes they do. So when we learn from another person's mistakes, or our own mistakes, we gain more discrimination about what is destructive for us and what is pointing us towards more healing. In other words, we effect a healing through our discrimination. We become more likely to choose what is positive for us rather than what is negative so we gain more joy, more light, and perpetuate that upward spiral of growth and increased consciousness.

Once we understand the mind, we will stop being ruled by it. When we come to the consciousness of accepting our pain, accepting the mistakes we have made, accepting our diseases, we will then stop being ruled by the diseases. We will stop being ruled by our own thoughts, our own attitudes and opinions, and our own reactions to everyone and everything around us. It is our own reactions that create the disharmonies and diseases in our lives.

Many of today's therapies teach us about the hate we have for our mothers and our fathers. They teach us to hate our parents for what they have done to us. We need to recognize that hate destroys. Hate is war and destruction. Most of all, hate destroys the hater. Hate creates disease in the one who hates. Forgiveness heals. Acceptance and forgiveness of ourselves and others reverses the disease process and creates a healing. The only way to begin this healing process is to take responsibility for our own thoughts, emotions, and attitudes.

When we truly accept that our own emotions are the cause of disease in our lives, then we will start treating those emotions that are around us as diseases. We will then know and understand that when someone is very angry we can catch that anger just like a cold. If we attach to the anger of another person, that anger will spread. So we learn to take precautions when it comes to dealing with other people's emotions as well as our own.

For example, hepatitis affects the liver and is a disease of anger, the fire. The vibration of anger is contagious and gets passed on from one person to another. Like attracts like whether positive or negative. This law of attraction explains how one group of people gets hepatitis while another group does not, even though everyone is drinking the same water and basically doing the same things. The disease comes from the amount of anger that people have in them. Certain people catch the same diseases due to the attachment that they have to each other's anger.

Similarly, cancer is a disease of attachment (the water) that has reached almost plague proportions in this country. Cancer begins at the emotional level with the stagnation of those emotions. Cancer is a toxic build-up in the emotions and in the body. The water principle in the body, which is the emotions, becomes putrid. Emotions have been stuffed and stored for so long that many cells of the body become negative. They grow and multiply until they dominate the positive, healthy cells. The soul says to the body, "Look, you've dumped enough negativity into me, it's time to check out. It's time to get rid of this body and go for a new one."

It's just like a diaper, really. When a baby fills up a diaper, we have to get rid of it. The same principle occurs within the body. When the toxicity from the emotions builds up, the body begins to rot. If we look at the body of a cancer victim, we can understand. The body stinks. The flesh, which is a combination of fear (earth) and attachment (water), is rotting. The emotions have been stuck, stagnant, and fermenting for so long that the body finally starts to reflect that inner emotional distress.

The disease of cancer is what happens when we are unable to accept the creative energy of the fire principle which is the masculine energy of responsibility, direction, knowledge, and experience. The masculine energy is authority; the authority in ourselves and in others. When we reject the masculine, creative energy, our fire principle gets blocked. The male fire cannot heat the feminine water, the emotions, to produce steam which keeps the elimination working in the body at all levels. When this blockage in the male energy happens, the negative female part of us runs away with itself.

What I want to get across is that we are constantly surrounded by disease: fear, attachment, anger, desire, and grief. There is no exit. We cannot go up into the Himalayas and escape from our emotions. We cannot go into the mountains, dig a cave, and forget about the five passions. We all have to go through these emotions as long as we are in a human body. It does not matter whether these emotions are outside or inside of our own minds. Thoughts or actions both boil down to the same energy.

By getting stuck in the pleasure-pain problem, we get stuck in our emotions. Seeking more and more pleasure is not the way to get rid of our pain. The only way to get rid of the pain is by going through it and then we will gain something very different from pleasure. We will come to know true joy and bliss.

Healing comes from the emotional attachment we have to the healer. We get healed not by anything in particular that the healer does but rather through the karma we have with the healer. If our karma is to heal, then we heal. This includes healing with a medical doctor or a natural physician. The healing depends on our karmas.

We are now moving from the Piscean Age, which is one of secretiveness, into the Aquarian Age, which is one of truth and openness. The nature of the Piscean energy is secretiveness. The Piscean gives to a few, while the Aquarian energy is truth-bearing and gives to many. Simultaneously, we are under the influence of a much longer time span which encompasses the transition from the Iron Age, which is one of mental consciousness, to the Golden Age, which is one of soul consciousness. We are actually dealing with two overlapping time periods which are affecting the evolution of human consciousness on our planet.

Right now, we are half-way through the Iron Age and we are feeling a great deal of pressure; there is a hell on earth. At the same time, we are also moving towards the Golden Age so we are feeling the influence of both periods. The Golden Age is a real polarity. As far as the mind goes, it is a great time because a lot of people have truth and understanding on the inside, while on the outside there is a lot of negativity and hell. The energy of the Golden Age is one that burns us in the hell that we create for ourselves.

If we work towards goodness and take responsibility for what we know and understand, our soul consciousness evolves. If we do not, the soul gets tortured. Since we are half-way through the Iron Age, we feel the hell that is building up on earth right now. Our soul does not need to be tortured as much since we are already being tortured by the state of the world around us.

The next part to understand is that detachment is healing. When we become detached we are healing. People often misunderstand detachment. They think that detachment means going up into the mountains by themselves and sitting there, year after year, with no thoughts or temptation from sex, alcohol, drugs or anything in the material world. People think if they stay in the mountains all their passions will disappear. This is total nonsense because when these people come down from the mountain their minds will immediately run wild and be pulled back to their old patterns.

I call these people the yogi types. They put up a wall and think it will protect them from their desires and emotions. What these people do not understand is that if we dam up a river and do not build an avenue for the water to run through, the dam will break down. The water will back up, and back up, until finally the whole structure collapses. So we need to put in a spillway, a hole in the dam. Instead of blocking all that power, we can put in a waterwheel and get energy from it.

We need to use the principle of the waterwheel when learning detachment from the emotions of this material plane. We need to learn how to switch all the power of our negativity, which is destroying us, into positivity and detachment, which will heal us. We need to re-direct our power. For example, we can take all the explosive sexual energy that we are scattering and use it for healing ourselves and others. We can direct that sexual energy towards generating more and more awareness, more vitality, less disease, and more physical and emotional elimination.

By re-directing our power into positivity, the mind becomes healthier and we have a heightened awareness about the different parts of our lives. We become more conscious of our emotions, our feelings, and our diseases. We start to be more conscious of our bodies and what is going on inside of them. We begin the lifelong process of bringing our body-mind into balance and we are able to live and love in accordance with our higher self, our soul, and the will of God.

As we become conscious of ourselves and our actions, we become more concentrated and focused. Then time and space become very different. Instead of speeding up, we are actually slowing down. We are not at the mercy of our emotions, which speed us up and cause disease. Each moment then becomes longer because we are more aware and less reactionary.

When we are concentrated and focused, we really experience the polarity of time and space. Time is motion, the male energy. The more conscious we are, the more space we create, the feminine energy. Time is always attracted to space. The catch is, time cannot fill all the space that is created by stilling the mind through concentration and focus. Time constantly keeps us moving.

As we become more conscious, we work towards being still. We practice stillness of mind. Stillness means the mind does not move at all. When we are emotional, we are very speedy. Speed is very quick time or motion. As we become less emotional and react less often, the actual time, in the space of our reactions, is taken up by our growing consciousness. Instead of reacting, we take the time to slow down and we respond instead of react. We go inside ourselves for the truth of the situation before we automatically react.

Most of the time we are numb. We say and do things totally from habit. That is the animal part of ourselves. We are constantly acting from the four lower chakras which contain the passions: desire, anger, love (attachment) and fear.

Very rarely do we stay in the ether, the throat chakra, where we feel the space, the grief, and the longing. When we are experiencing that grief and longing, then our vision becomes clear. We know the truth. The ether (space) is the highest emotion in the human body because when it is used positively, the longing leads us to the Lord, to the soul, to our spiritual nature. When we feel the space, when we are in our grief, we have the opportunity to act spontaneously from our soul quality.

When we really become one-pointed in our lives, we are dealing with the principle of homeopathy; that is, a little bit goes a long way. A small act can have a profound effect. When we are paying attention to what we are saying and doing, we are able to go upwards away from the fear, attachment, anger, and desire, and straight to the ether. There, in the ether, we are able to experience the positivity of our space. We feel the nothingness and that feeling helps us to be receptive. This receptivity is what nature is all about. Nature is a mother, the earth. She is

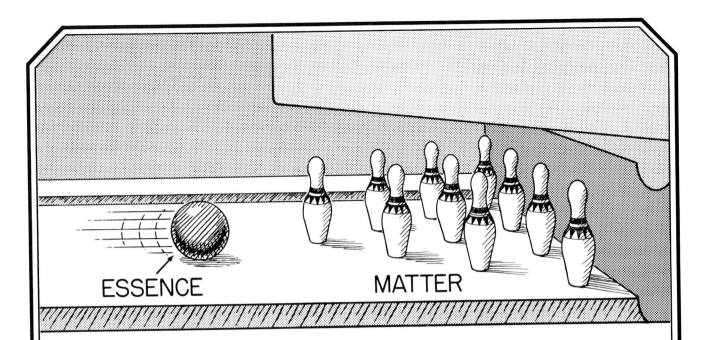

ESSENCE　　　　MATTER

The Homeopathic Principle

"A little bit goes a long way." Homeopathy uses a single
vibrational *essence* to effect a change in the energy state of the
whole person. Using bowling as an analogy, it takes one ball in
the right place to knock down all of the pins.

receptive to heaven, to the power of the creative, to that
fiery energy.

So as we slow down, we have opportunities to become
more conscious, to learn, to accept, and to dig deeply
within ourselves. We can learn what is coming in the
future by looking at the past. The past is where we can see
our mistakes and the mistakes of our parents. Those mistakes show us where the energy is blocked. By recognizing
those mistakes, we have an opportunity for rebirth, for
growth. This growth will happen if we look at those mistakes and learn from them.

So by looking at our past, we see how our present is
the blueprint of our future. As we take advantage of what

our past has taught us, we experience the now. We experience the present because the present is conscious. When we are not at the mercy of our emotions, we are in the present, we are totally conscious, and time stands still. Then we experience everything so deeply that days feel like months, and months become years. We begin to experience nothingness. This does not mean we live forever, it means we gain an understanding of where the idea of forever comes from.

I've spent some time in India, and the people there have an understanding of their relationship to their parents and how they are attached to their mothers and fathers. They also understand how that attachment gets passed on from generation to generation.

There are places in India where I've seen very negative situations, where there is a lot of poverty, and yet within the families there is still a tremendous amount of love and vitality. This polarity exists because, if there's one law that fits this creation it is, "Where there is the most resistance there is the most energy." If we have a dam, and we make a pathway for the water to flow through, we can generate a great amount of energy. When the resistance behind the dam is channeled, it turns into power, and that power can light up cities. That same power can literally lighten us up, lighten our load.

In the midst of all the poverty I saw in India, I also saw an incredible vital energy. What I'm talking about is the vibration, the nature of mind in India. The Indian mind does not have the meat-eater's vibration. In India it is vegetarian or non-vegetarian. Here in America we are meat eaters or non-meat eaters. The mental waves are very different. The vibration in India is very, very accepting. The vibration in the United States is very, very threatening.

I often get the question from students, "This Alive Polarity program is so wonderful. How do I function in the outside world when I leave here?" What I tell them is, there is no such thing as the outside world. The "outside world" is everything that we look at outside of ourselves. The real question is, "How do I create what I feel is positive, which is outside of me right now, outside of me all the time?" I tell people that the trick is to attract to themselves all the time the same likeness they are feeling right now. In other words, all the positivity they feel when they ask this question will be repeated everywhere they go, because positivity on the inside is always reflected on the outside. Then, even in a negative situation we are able to find what is positive.

So what I am saying is we get drawn to whatever energy we manifest. By developing our sensitivity and cleaning up our body-mind, we attract higher and higher vibrations to ourselves. This process of cleansing takes time. When this cleansing comes it is wonderful, truly wonderful.

It actually takes at least twelve years to clean out all the actions we have done in the past which have moved us towards the negative. To cleanse the body completely takes at least seven years of being a strict vegetarian. Then, in addition to that cleansing of our physical body, we need to work on each of the five emotions (elements) of fear (earth), attachment (water), anger (fire), desire (air), and grief (ether), for another five years. A full purification takes at least twelve years, the entire cycle of the zodiac; one year for every sign of the zodiac. Then we really start getting tuned up. We start to be truly alive.

What we are doing in the Alive Fellowship is creating the higher vibration of the East, the consciousness of the vegetarian, as a teaching model for regeneration in the West. We are teaching about vibration in a form that is comprehensible to Westerners. We are learning to live in the West with the soul consciousness of the East, which means having the understanding that every living thing has a soul. We are learning to think and act from our higher selves so that we can live with a silver spoon in our mouths and not be attached to it. I would rather be born in the East as a vegetarian, totally poverty-stricken, with nothing, than be a rich person with a silver spoon in my mouth and eat meat until I die.

In order to understand the specifics of disease and emotion, we must come to a point where we will take a risk, where we will let ourselves become vulnerable and take a chance. At that time, we need to use all our human discrimination, choose what course we will take, and establish the priorities in our lives. Then we become the fool and take the leap off the mountain. Everyone around us will see us as a fool because of their own attachments, their own diseases, and their own emotions. If we take the leap that means they are going to take the leap too, some-day, because of their attachment to us. As we go through the process of becoming more conscious and breaking old family patterns, at first our parents are fearful as they watch us make the jump.

That leap, that step, is a step we all must take. The key

is, we must learn to take that step more than once because we will all take that step when we die. So the thing to do is to start developing our discrimination. Then we will know how and when to take that step towards greater consciousness and we will take it before we die. When we use our discrimination to take positive steps, we make ourselves vulnerable to the consequences. When we take responsibility for our own choices and accept what comes back to us, we become vulnerable and we have the power. We are receptive.

It was a big leap for me when I decided I would remain celibate until I got married. Celibacy was a very big step for me because I have a lot of sexual energy. Even though I felt very much like a fool I knew it was the right thing to do. I became vulnerable to people's criticism since celibacy was not in fashion in the early seventies. Out of this leap, and the willingness to be vulnerable, has come the tremendous positivity of my marriage and the power of the Fellowship.

In the Alive Fellowship we teach people how to use their sexual energy positively for healing instead of scattering their sexual energy and dissipating it. We teach people how to focus all their sexual energy in a committed marriage relationship or remain unmarried and celibate. Sexual energy is attraction, magnetism, and emotional attachment. At the Fellowship, the energy of emotional attachment is used positively to develop consciousness and promote healing. The healing energy at the Alive Fellowship pulls many people to do their work on themselves.

After all, we have to look at our own lives. I think we

all know when and where we have taken great leaps. I'm talking about the times we really felt like a fool and people laughed and made fun of us. I know that some people come to the Alive Polarity programs and their friends really give them a hard time. Their friends are still taking cocaine and dope and sleeping around. At the same time, they are really feeling a pull because they are attached to the people who come here. When we take a positive, conscious step, we take our family and friends with us because they are holding on to us. Meanwhile, they are all saying, "Whoa!" because they know what is in store for them. So either they have to let go, which is very painful, or they go with the pull.

Any person who has made a significant contribution to humanity on this planet, who has a high level of consciousness, has had to take these leaps. Every person on this earth has the potential and ability to be a humanitarian. It all depends on our attachments, on whom we picked for our parents and whether we reject or accept them. How we use our discrimination now is what is important.

We need to learn to stop condemning and start accepting. We must have the courage to make mistakes and accept mistakes as part of the whole process. If we learn from those mistakes, we will become more and more conscious. The healing process will continue. If we do not learn, and we repeat the same mistakes, our life lessons will become more and more intense, more and more tamasic or scattered, until we get the message. Our life will become like a train that has picked up speed and momentum and is almost impossible to stop.

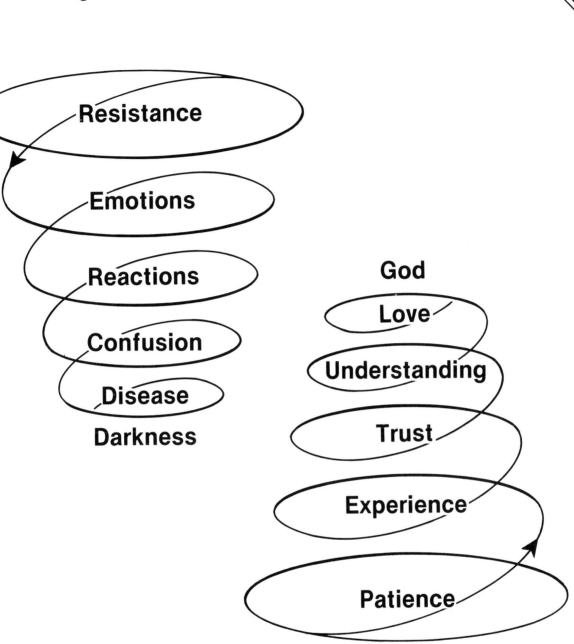

Resistance

Emotions

Reactions

Confusion

Disease

Darkness

God

Love

Understanding

Trust

Experience

Patience

Fundamental Choices

Free will is the attitude we choose towards the events that come to us.
Our destiny unfolds according to our past actions and choices. If we
make negative choices in our attitudes now, we will create a downward
spiral of disease in our lives. If we make positive choices in our attitudes,
we perpetuate an upward spiral of growth and healing.

When consciousness gets a foothold, the healing starts to happen. When our discrimination develops to the point of being able to choose positive situations for ourselves rather than destructive ones, the body-mind goes through a healing crisis. When we are healing, the energy in the body-mind moves through at an increased rate. The negativity stored inside of us gets pushed out. The negativity surfaces and an elimination takes place.

Mentally, emotionally, and physically the toxins will leave us. The weight of negativity cannot stay in us anymore as our vibration increases. The deadness cannot exist as we become more conscious and more alive, so that deadness, that negative matter, leaves. The drugs we took, the novocaine, the aspirin, the acid, the cocaine, the nicotine, the marijuana, and the alcohol, cannot stay inside us any longer. The lust, the greed, the pride, the attachment, the fear, the desire, and the anger all start to drop away as we cleanse our body-mind in our quest for healing.

Now, at the moments when these negative agents are leaving us, at whatever level they are eliminating, we will experience a time of transition. As the negativity surfaces, we will experience a test, because very likely we will feel physical, mental, and emotional anxiety and a desire for the very things we are on the verge of eliminating.

One day, after I had been a vegetarian a while, I experienced just such a test. I had been lying down for a short time and all of a sudden I felt stoned, not only stoned, but the most intensely stoned I had ever been. Even though I had only smoked a small amount of marijuana in my life, it had accumulated in my body. At that moment, I wanted to go out and say, "Hey, roll me one will you?"

You see, I was experiencing the same energy I felt when I smoked marijuana. I was eliminating, so the same symptoms were coming to the surface. The key moment comes when the elimination takes place. Then we have to decide whether to take the toxins back into ourselves or to be conscious and refuse to give in to the negativity. This key moment is when our discrimination comes into play.

Once we have gone through a healing crisis, especially with things like drugs, cigarettes, and alcohol, we become very sensitive because of the depth of the cleansing. We can be fifty feet from someone and know if they have been smoking cigarettes or if they have been drinking alcohol. Our body just tightens up and groans because it knows what is going on.

Remember the first time we smoked a cigarette? We choked on the smoke and felt like we were going to die. We thought, "My God, people are crazy for smoking. This is terrible." Then later, because of peer group pressure, we started smoking. We thought, "Oh, smoking is so 'in'. I want to be grown up and be like everyone else."

If we were lucky at the time, we had the awareness that the people who smoked were grown-up and that they were sick, and we did not want to be sick. Or we got so sick from smoking the cigarettes we said, "I don't care how grown up this is supposed to be, I'm sick and I don't want to be sick, so forget it!" We might have had enough of an impression from a past life, when we died of lung cancer or whatever the disease, that we immediately rejected the cigarettes, alcohol, or drugs.

So we become the person who drives home from the party when everyone else is too drunk. Or, if we have not made the switch, we become the person who drives home drunk; so drunk we drive off a cliff and for some reason survive. That is when we realize we are killing ourselves. Though, instead of killing ourselves, we live and are able to say, "No more. I will not drink anymore. I almost killed myself. In fact I should have killed myself and I don't even understand the reason I didn't kill myself. Therefore, I am going to stop drinking and I will face the feelings and the issues that are causing me to drink, causing me to want to numb myself." So we stop drinking and find out the root of our drinking problem. This life-death situation is a great gift. It is a transition point, a chance for rebirth.

Very often we have a physical elimination after we have experienced mental and emotional awareness. One day I was teaching a class on the manipulations we use in our Alive Polarity energy balancing sessions. There was a person in the class who belonged to Alcoholics Anonymous. He was about fifty years old and a leader in the organization. For the last twenty years he had sworn he would not drink. Every day he said, "I won't drink. I'm happy and I'm free." I was attempting to teach him that as long as the thoughts about alcohol were still there, the desire for the alcohol and the alcohol itself were still in his body. He was skeptical.

During the class I was working on a twenty-two year old boy using manipulations to get his energy moving. The boy was learning about becoming a man. I leaned over his shoulders and worked on his scapula and diaphragm. Then I began to press on his liver. As I increased the movement of energy in his body, his vibration increased. The negativity could not stay in his body any longer and an elimination occurred. He began to reek of alcohol. The smell was of a "pure grade" whiskey.

I motioned to the fifty year old man and said, "Come here, I want to teach you something. I have just increased the energy in this man's body and I want you to put your nose close to his mouth as he breathes. This man hasn't had a drink for six months."

The ex-alcoholic said, "I believe you. I haven't seen him drinking around here." Then he bent over the man and took a whiff. He almost passed out. The smell of alcohol made him stagger backwards, and with his eyes closed he said, "Jack Daniels, my favorite drink." Right after that statement the twenty-two year old said, "Jack Daniels is all I ever drank since I was fourteen."

So the fifty year old man realized that he needed to do some work on himself. He needed to do emotional awareness work on being an alcoholic. He needed to face what it was that he got from drinking even though he knew it was a very negative thing to do. So along with the awareness work, proper diet, fasting, sessions, and exercises he gained more consciousness, and sure enough he started to eliminate.

When we begin to do our work, the mental, emotional, and physical negativity all eliminate together. We can usually accept the physical elimination that happens through the body. We begin to feel cleaner and purer as our vibration increases and gets higher. We don't eat meat anymore, we don't drink or take drugs, we focus our sexual energy in a committed marriage, or we are celibate. Sometimes we even get a little cocky about how pure we think we are.

But, when it comes to an emotional elimination it's often another story. We usually don't want to accept our reactions. When we eliminate through the emotions, all the negativity, all the ugliness of our fears, our attachments, our anger, our desires, and our grief comes to the surface. We are able to see, feel, and hear all the emotions that we have stuffed and stored over the years; all the feelings that caused our initial desire to numb ourselves will surface.

When an emotional elimination of this kind occurs, it is the most important time to have courage, to be an observer and realize that these emotions are not ours. These emotions belong to the mind, not to the soul. By keeping in mind that the soul is really happy about the elimination process, we can accept our emotions and then let go of them. We will all go through some emotional reactions. What we need to understand is that the emotional reactions will occur less and less as we become more and more conscious. Real consciousness comes from truly letting go of the emotional reactions that have been fed into us through our attachments to our mothers and fathers and to their mothers and fathers.

As we raise our vibration, our consciousness grows, and our attachments to our parents change. We pull our parents instead of our parents pulling us. In other words, instead of reacting to our parents, our parents react to us. Our parents will go through their emotions and they will have to deal with them. Their emotions will not be ours anymore. Thank the Lord!

Like attracts like. Instead of our likeness pulling us

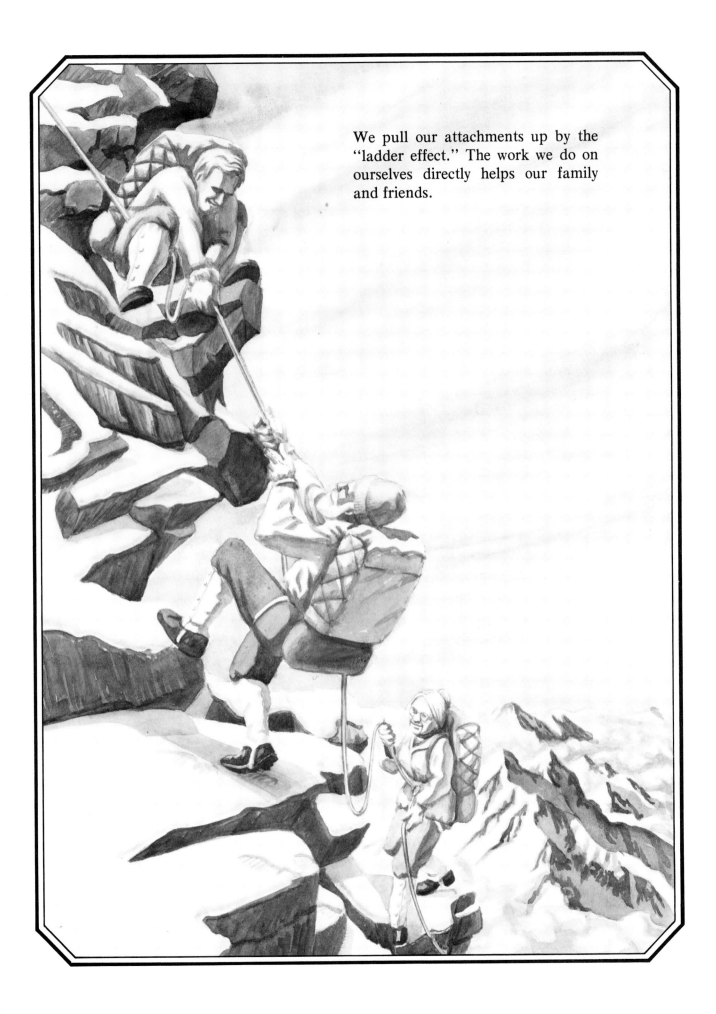

We pull our attachments up by the "ladder effect." The work we do on ourselves directly helps our family and friends.

down to a grosser vibration, our likeness can pull us up to a higher, finer vibration. This pulling power is especially obvious when it comes to our attachments to our parents. We become a mirror for our parents; when they look at us they see themselves, the positivity and the negativity. Our parents start looking at themselves, questioning themselves, and growing from the reflection we are giving them. They also become a mirror for us. They can mirror our positivity as well as our negativity. They become a reflection of our own energy.

My father, for example, is actually feeling the energy of the Alive Fellowship and the work we are doing here. He does not really understand what I am doing and yet emotionally he is very happy. He used to drink a lot and now he drinks very little because he feels the healing energy coming from me, his attachment. He has big earlobes, lots of vitality, and he is rebounding back. My mom is now attempting to catch up with him, whereas before, she was the one who had more vitality.

What I am talking about is a "ladder effect." We pull each other up the ladder by our reflection, by the energy bouncing off of us. Gaining this reflective ability is like putting wax on a car. When water (emotions) hits the wax, the water beads up, rolls off, and does not hurt the finish.

When we come to understand consciousness, and the process of accepting our particular attachments to our parents, we also accept the diseases they have in their lives. Through this acceptance we immediately accept our own diseases. We stop "should-ing" our parents. We stop saying, "You should do this and you should do that."

Instead, "We do this and we do that." We are the doers. Instead of their vibration and their attachment destroying us, our vibration and our healing starts to affect them.

The attraction to our parents that originally drew us to them (our original polarity) is pulled upward and inward, and the negativity that has been destroying us is now turned into power, energy, and healing. That power heals our relationships, it heals our bodies, it heals our parents' bodies, and it heals the bodies of future generations.

As our energy moves inward rather than outward, we return to our emotional base and to the energies that were weaving us at the time of conception. We move back up into the ether. We move back inward to where we started. Our descent into this creation is reversed and we move upward through the chakras: from the earth, to the water, to the fire, to the air, to the ether. We move upward from the fear, to the attachment, through the anger, to the desire, until we reach the grief and experience the longing.

In the ether we gain the skill of discrimination. We learn from our parents' mistakes and accept their energy inside us, in our blood. We learn from our own mistakes and start detaching from our parents and attaching to God. Attaching to God is our only security. We move from our parents to God, to the Lord, to the Oneness. By understanding the polarities that exist we move toward union. This work is the power of Alive Polarity.

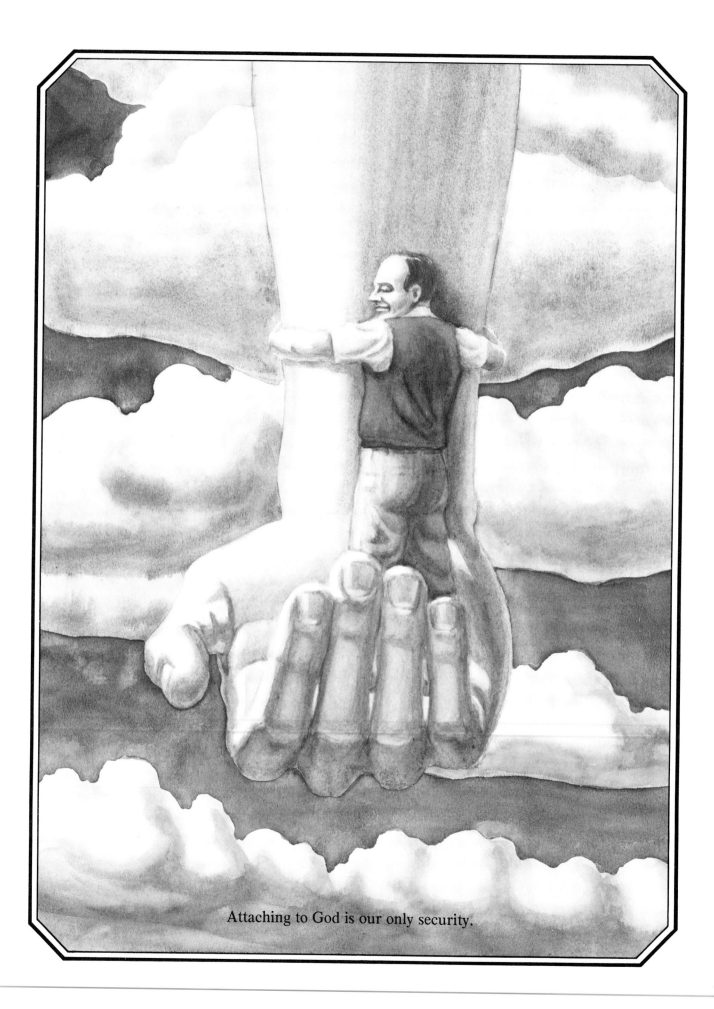

Attaching to God is our only security.

VI

Life Cycles from Conception to Death:
Awareness through Life Histories

In the beginning is life. In the end is death. For every beginning there is an end because this earth is a world of duality, of polarity. Within one end of the spectrum lies the potential, the seed, of the other. We are literally born to die. Our whole life is a preparation for our death. How we live our life will be how we die. If we are in misery our whole life, we will die with great pain. If we are positive and conscious, we will die with a look of serenity on our face.

Briefly, there are four cycles or periods of life in this human body. The first period is from conception to the age of thirteen, when we start to become an adult. It is a time of exploration and learning.

The second time period runs from thirteen to twenty-eight. During this second period we become mature adults. We come to terms with what it means to be a householder: being part of a family, finding a job, and learning what it is like to have and raise children.

The third period runs from thirty to about fifty-five or sixty years old. This is a time period for completing the family and being grandparents. It is a period when we have complete authority within the family. We are respected as the teacher. Through our experience of being an adult and raising children, we gain a tremendous amount of experience and wisdom in the world. We are not only the teachers within our nuclear family, we are teachers of the extended human family as well.

The fourth stage is from about sixty-five to when we die. This is a time when we can relax from our worldly responsibilities and let them fall upon the shoulders of our children. Our entire attention can now be focused on our union with God. It is a time of completion for our spiritual life, when we make final preparations to die into oneness with the Lord.

I. Conception to age Thirteen:
A time of exploration and learning.

II. Fourteen to Twenty-Eight:
Becoming mature adults and learning to be householders.

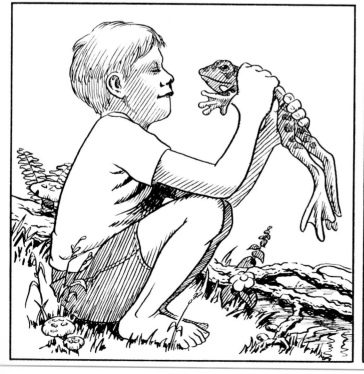

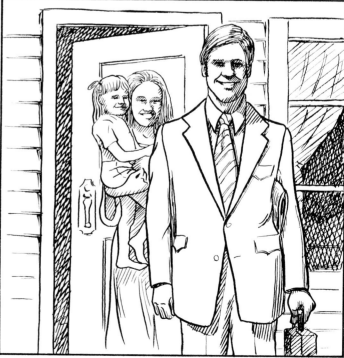

It is interesting to note here that the length of our sleep time changes throughout these cycles to accommodate the learning processes that are taking place. Young children sleep many, many hours. As we progress through the second stage, we sleep eight to ten hours depending on our individual make-up. As we get older and older, God seems to allow for less and less sleep, until we get to a point where we are sixty-five or seventy and sleep only three or four hours a night.

In our society we give older people tranquilizers to make them sleep instead of encouraging them to utilize their extra waking time in a constructive and positive way. The same misunderstanding is reflected in the effort by old people in America to look and dress like teenagers. Old age is not appreciated or encouraged in this culture as a treasured time to be in the world and prepare for death, which is a wonderful experience. During this time the

III. Twenty-Eight to Fifty-Six: Gaining authority and experience in the world, teaching what we have learned.

IV. Fifty-Six to Death: Having wisdom, completing our spiritual life and preparing for death.

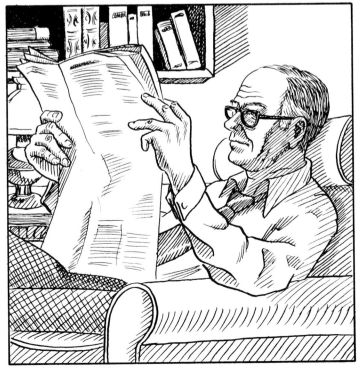

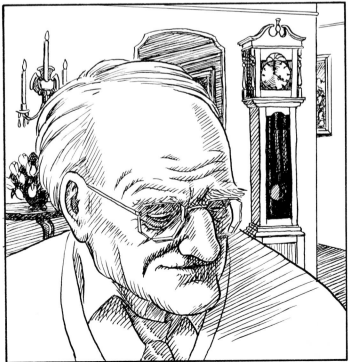

Lord is preparing us to meditate, to look inward instead of outward, which reverses the habit of a lifetime.

A good friend of mine had a grandmother who was not sleeping. His grandmother no longer wanted to take the sleeping pills the doctor had prescribed. He told her, "Grandma, forget the sleeping pills. Don't take them. When you wake up after your three hours of sleep, get into your rocking chair, close your eyes, and meditate. Just be with yourself and feel your presence with God."

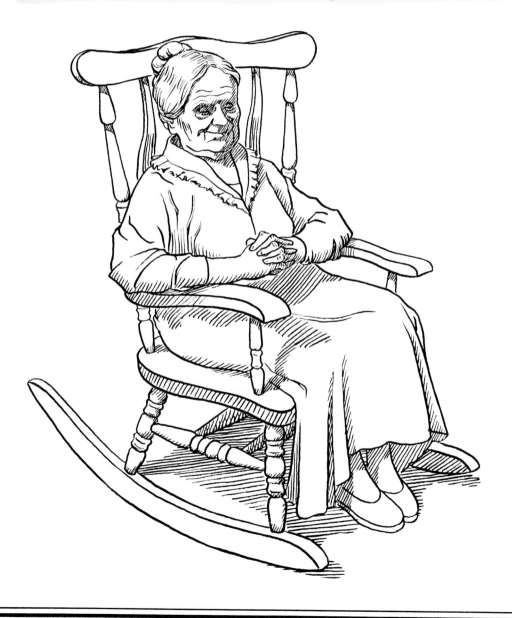

His grandmother has been meditating ever since. She has become very happy instead of very sad and depressed as she had been. She has gotten closer and closer to God and has become very serene about dying.

When we are young our main thrust is outward into the world. We do not want to think about dying. As we get older we accept our responsibility to go home to the Lord. We look forward to the time of our death as another of life's transitions, another rite of passage in the transformation of our human consciousness.

We can help our consciousness to grow and expand by developing understanding and awareness. Awareness can occur to us at any moment and in many ways. One of the most powerful tools for cultivating awareness is examining the patterns that repeat themselves throughout our life history. The patterns in our life history will show us either our negativity (where we are stuck, where our blocks are), or our positivity (where there is the most movement and growth). A life history gives us an overview. It is a map that shows how our specific mind patterns can manifest from our birth to our death.

Particularly during the major transitions in our lives, we are given an opportunity to see very clearly, very graphically, who we are and how we react. In the East these transitions are defined according to life cycles: conception, birth, childhood, adulthood, and the time period at the end of our lives when we prepare for death by going inside and focusing on God. It is the knowledge we gain by going through each of these transitions that gives us the consciousness to be in harmony with our soul's destiny.

Astrologically, these life cycle transitions occur approximately every fourteen years, beginning at our birth and following consecutively until our death. These key points are when Saturn, the planet of discipline and limitation, the tester, the Lord of Karma, is either in opposition to the position it had in the heavens at the time of our birth, or has returned to that original position. What this astrological movement means for us is that Saturn is teaching us our life lessons by making them

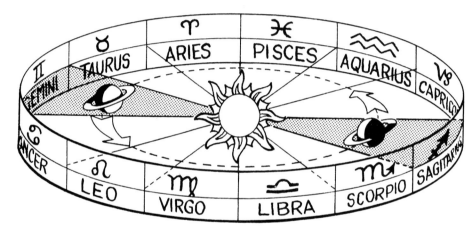

"Saturn Oppositions" and "Saturn Returns"

Saturn takes approximately twenty-nine years to orbit the sun and traverse the zodiac. So, every fourteen years we are either experiencing a "Saturn Opposition" or a "Saturn Return." A "Saturn Opposition" means that Saturn has moved into the sign that is the exact opposite (180 degrees) to the sign Saturn resided in at our birth. For example, if we are born with Saturn in the sign of Sagittarius, it will move into the sign of Gemini when we are approximately fourteen. When we reach the age of approximately twenty-eight, we experience what is commonly referred to as the "Saturn Return." At this time, Saturn is in the same position as it was at our birth, or conjunct to our natal Saturn.

The "Saturn Opposition" and the "Saturn Return" are opportunities to see our negative patterns more intensely, in situations that may be very painful, and then choose a positive and healing course of action rather than continuing in a negative and destructive way.

more acute and more visible during these transition times in our lives.

Our life lessons will be emphasized at these transitions, especially if we have not been doing the work we need to do on ourselves all along the way. By understanding what is occurring at these transition times, we can become more aware of situations that are repeating themselves and we can learn to discriminate which ones are good for us and which ones are destructive.

These transitions begin at conception, they begin with what was happening between our parents at that time. The next key point is our birth, and again at ages 14, 28, 42, 56, 70, and 84. What we do or do not do at these transitions determines how our lives will continue to unfold.

What we need to understand is that we are here in this world to do certain work on ourselves. Astrologically, Saturn is showing us the lessons we need to learn so we may fully develop ourselves as human beings. Our lives will become more and more tamasic (or scattered), more and more sour, if we miss what is being shown to us during these key periods. On the other hand, if we do see our negative patterns and are able to reverse them by a conscious effort, then we can begin an upward spiral of growth and positive change.

An example of how we can sustain and enhance the positivity in our life history can be illustrated by some of my patterns since my birth. I was born to an English mother who gave me up for adoption at birth. Essentially, this was a very courageous choice for her to make. She decided to put me up for adoption so I could enter an environment with parents who really wanted a child and had the means to support one.

When I reached fourteen, this same courage and positivity was repeated. I was in the eighth grade and was becoming a young man. It was then that I was picked from my football team, the La Morinda Thunderbirds, to be on the All-Star "Pop Warner" team called the East Bay All-Stars; "Pop Warner" is like a Little League for older kids.

I was a white, rich kid on a mostly lower class, mostly black All-Star team. At first, all the black kids hated my guts because of the polarities of black-white and rich-poor. They continually tested me. They would pick on me and hit me in the groin in a tackle. Even so, in one-on-one tackling I was able to break through the line by plowing through head first. They did not expect that of me. By being gutsy, playing really hard, taking risks, and being responsible, I gave the team everything I had. By the end of the practice week I had won the respect of everyone on the team. The energy switched from hate to love, they made me a co-captain of the All-Star team, and we all played well together.

When I turned twenty-eight I was in the midst of combining my knowledge of various teachings in order to create the Alive Fellowship as a form for Alive Polarity. The lesson for me at this time was to continue the upward spiral of positivity that began with my mother's decision to give me up to a solid family when I was born. At fourteen and at twenty-eight I was able to have the courage to acknowledge and take responsibility for myself as a leader and a teacher. So by looking at my life history we can see how my positive actions at fourteen, when I was becoming an adult, were stepped up in vibration when I turned twenty-eight, the time of mature adulthood.

Our positivity or negativity intensifies depending upon whether or not we do the work on ourselves that helps our consciousness to evolve. This transformative process is how we learn. Our freedom from destructive situations comes from wanting to do what needs to be done in order for our higher and lower selves to be in harmony.

The life history of a man named Paul, who came to see me when he was fifty-six, is a good example of how negativity can intensify when feelings are not dealt with as they come up. His daughter, Sarah, was twenty-eight and she had just been diagnosed as having cancer.

As Paul recounted his life history to me, he said that his brother, David, had also gotten cancer at twenty-eight and died. He told me that from the time that he and his brother were born, until the time they were fourteen, their mother and grandmother fought constantly. It turned out that David became more upset and more strongly attached to the negativity of his mother and grandmother's fighting than did his brother Paul. So the cancer, the negativity, was really "caught" when David was fourteen. Since the feelings that came up during David's first life cycle had not been resolved, his feelings manifested as a physical disease at the next transition period when he was twenty-eight.

Paul then told me that his daughter, Sarah, was born when he turned twenty-eight. Now, at fifty-six, Paul saw that his unresolved negative emotions had been passed on to his daughter who, at twenty-eight, was manifesting the same family disease at exactly the same transition point when her uncle died and at the age when her father and mother conceived her.

This family history shows how patterns are passed on from generation to generation. I hope it gives each of us the impetus to express our feelings and clear up our fears and confusions. By resolving our negativities, we are able to pass on positive patterns to our children and their children. The work we are doing on ourselves is really secondary. Primarily, we are becoming clear for the benefit of future generations.

In order for us to understand our patterns, or "family diseases," we need to realize fully what it means to be a human being in all our stages from conception until our death. When we recognize and accept the teaching of our life cycles, we can start to take responsibility for the consciousness we have as human beings.

So let's examine conception as a point in time when we as souls come into this world of time and space. At the moment of conception, through the reaction of the sperm of our father exploding into the egg of our mother, the soul consciously incarnates. Through this attachment to our parents and the work we need to do with them in our lives, we are able to use their vitality to become a physical body.

When the body-mind has been fully created, three months after birth, we will have passed through the entire twelve-month cycle of the zodiac, from Aries to Pisces. Each sign of the zodiac governs the development of some part of the body-mind. So we really take twelve months to fully develop from head to foot rather than the accepted

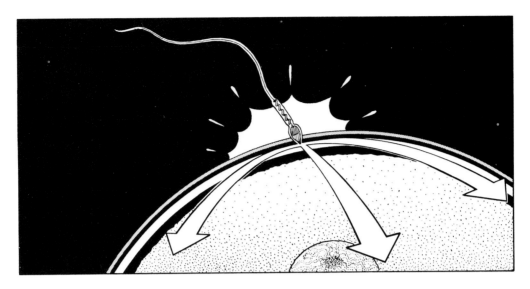

From the point on the egg where the sperm makes contact,
a dramatic and exceedingly fast wave-like reaction spreads
in all directions around the egg.

nine-month cycle from conception to birth.

After we have completed our first twelve-month cycle of growth, we have a certain amount of vitality left over from the vitality our parents passed on to us for incarnation. Vitality is the magnetism that pulls together the sperm and the egg. The reaction makes a baby. It takes a great deal of vitality for a soul to conceive itself as a whole human being. If the quality of the vitality passed on by the parents is low, then their children will have a low reservoir of vitality from which to draw for the rest of their lives. If the quality of the parents' vitality is high, then less of this vitality will be needed for the conception and development of the organism, and the amount left over for the new human being will be higher.

Our vitality depends upon the quality of the vitality our parents passed on to us at conception. When parents are youthful, when they are mentally, emotionally, and physically healthy, they have a great deal of vitality to pass on to their children. But, if the parents are older, say thirty-eight, and have abused their bodies by squandering energy in having indiscriminate sex, using drugs, playing with psychic energy, drinking heavily, smoking cigarettes, or being trapped in negative thoughts and emotions, then the quality of the vitality their children receive will be low and depleted. The incoming soul will need to use a tremendous amount of the parents' vital energy to incarnate because the quality of the energy being passed on is not very strong.

This low vital energy situation can be reversed if parents who have abused themselves decide to change their consciousness before conceiving a child. Let's say they consciously conserve their energies and choose to remain celibate, or focus only on each other sexually, while they also do consistent work to re-build their bodies and minds. Then, after a few years, depending on the magnitude of their depletion, they will be able to pass on a much greater quality of vitality to their children. The conception will happen during a positive phase when they have been doing good things in their lives. Children conceived under these conditions have a greater vitality than their parents.

Vital energy is the foundation of how we are able to function and grow within the space suits we have been given for life on this earth. If we have high vitality, then we will be able to rebound faster from negative situations, whether they are physical, mental, or emotional. The healing process will work first with the reservoir of vital energy before it begins to drain the daily energy from the body and mind. This difference can be seen in the reactions of people who take lots of drugs. Some people can handle the drugs without a terrific reaction, while others cannot. People with low vitality really need to build up their energy and purify themselves in order to help mend their bodies, minds and emotions. If they do not apply this understanding and they follow a down-and-out cycle, be it with drugs, emotional stress, or by attracting accidents, their systems will be set on self-destruct and these people may die prematurely.

There are two aspects to vitality in the human body-mind. The first aspect is the vitality of the brain. This vitality determines how conscious we are able to be in the actions we do in the world. This conscious action comes from the fire principle through the umbilical current. Symbolically, this consciousness is depicted as a halo in pictures of saints. This vitality is measured by the length of the earlobes. Pictures of Gautama the Buddha often portray him as having very large earlobes and an expanded center of energy in his belly.

Large earlobes indicate a person's potential and ability to grow in consciousness quickly, in great leaps. A person with small earlobes will take more time. Big earlobes indicate an ability to recognize truth and and consciousness when it comes in front of us. We will easily recognize the truth of the lessons we need to learn. We will be able to go through the difficult or negative times in our lives and come out on the other side with a new understanding. Transformation will be easier.

Small earlobes indicate less of an ability to see consciousness and positivity in our lives. Our discrimination in making choices will be clouded. People who have small earlobes often need their life situations to become very tamasic, very heavy-handed and painful, before they are able to switch and see what is conscious and positive for them.

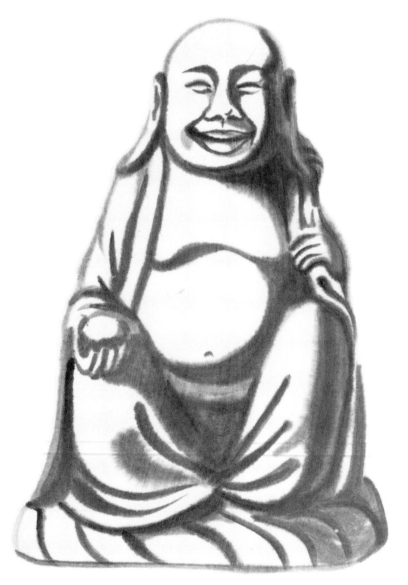

Buddha's large earlobes indicate a great
reservoir of vitality or consciousness.

The second aspect of human vitality is directed toward rebuilding the body. This vitality is specifically for the regeneration of cells in the body and comes from the water principle, or the sexual energy. This energy is centered in the pelvic area. The indicator of a greater or lesser degree of vitality in this area is the firmness of the buttocks. If the buttocks are flaccid and hang down like a curtain, the vitality of the parents was weak at the time of conception. What this weakness means for the child is that the cells will not be able to regenerate quickly and that healing, in general, will be slower.

What is important here is that we are dealing with the vitality of both the mental and the physical bodies. Some of us are given strong bodies, while others are given certain handicaps. These handicaps do not mean that both types cannot achieve the same success. It means that the ones with less vitality need to work harder to attain the same results.

So, at conception, we take on our parents' vitality quotient. We also take on our mother's and our father's characteristics as well as their attachments to their mothers and fathers. During the time period after conception until birth, we are the most attached we will ever be to our mother and father because through our mother we are constantly receiving both parents' emotions and reactions to the world. Still, the emphasis is on the direct relationship between the mother and the child she is carrying in her womb. The father's emotional patterns are passed on to the child through the mother by her emotional response to the father. It is through the mother's attachment to the father that the child picks up the father's specific emotional patterns. The manner in which the mother and father deal with each other's emotions, and the nature of their attachments in the world, will be reflected in the types of attitudes the new mind will project, as well as the structural form the new body will take.

Therefore, our internal human qualities are impressed upon us during this time. What happens during our stay inside the womb, from the moment of conception to the moment of birth, determines the blueprint for how we react for the rest of our lives. When we take our first

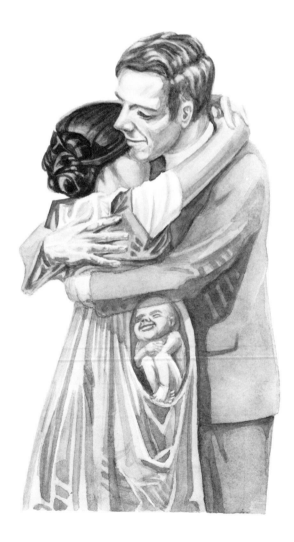

A father's emotional patterns are passed on to the child through the mother by her emotional response to the father.

breath, the air moves our energy outward. At that moment, the planetary positions make an imprint of how our inner patterns will manifest through our actions in this world. These actions may be read in our astrological chart.

The death of my brother, Peter, is a perfect example of how parents pass on their own imbalances and diseases to their children. Peter died of cancer at the age of two, making space for me to be adopted. For many years after my adoption, I prayed to Peter every night to thank him for giving me the opportunity to be accepted into such a loving family. As time went on I became attached to my mother's desire to know why Peter had died at such a young age. When I felt secure enough in my knowledge, I went to my mom and asked if she was ready to hear my explanation of Peter's early death. She said she was, so I fulfilled the desire she had since I first knew her. I gave her a way to understand what had happened to her son and what part she and her husband had played.

When my parents had D.B., my older brother, they were financially secure. They had a home and were very happy together. Two years later the war came and my father had to leave my mother. He had been in the war for about two years when he was badly injured in the leg. He was hospitalized for a year and had a big problem with the arteries and blood flow in his leg, as well as with the blood flow back to his heart. His blood vessels, a part of the creative male energy, were weak. When he got out of the hospital, he started drinking and taking lots of prescribed tranquilizers. He was very nervous and frustrated; he felt powerless.

It was during this time period that my parents decided to have another child and that child turned out to be Peter. The conception of Peter was very weak. The diseases and imbalances of my father that had to do with war, destruction, frustration, powerlessness, and a blood problem were passed on to Peter.

When my father returned from the war, physically and emotionally devastated, my mother's feelings and emotions were worry and fear. My understanding is that worry and fear are emotions that cause cancer. Peter died at the age of two because that was how long he could live in a body conceived from a father with weak male energy and a mother with worry and resentment.

I told my mother that cancer comes from a watery imbalance in our emotions. It comes from an inability to be in a cyclic form of flexibility. The receptive feminine energy, the water, is out of balance. I shared with her that from that time period of difficulty, she had held on to a great deal of pain and anguish.

It is interesting to me that since sharing this understanding with my mother, her attitude has slowly changed. Previously, both mom and dad had been to many doctors, searching everywhere for an answer. My mom said she felt my sincerity and that my explanation was unique. She could not be sure it was the truth, but since that time I have noticed that my mother is not as resentful as she used to be and she has cut down on her complaining about my dad. Generally, she is learning to be more receptive and supportive of my dad and me. My father, in turn, has stopped taking tranquilizers and is no longer drinking nearly as much as he used to. (It helped, too, that I gave him five cases of a non-alcoholic malt beverage for his birthday. This present was a positive and practical way to show my love for him and help him cut down on his alcohol intake.) Now, he is much happier and more creative. Through my mother's receptivity and understanding their relationship is healing.

This story illustrates how the relationship of the parents affects the conception of their child. Whether the child is strong or weak depends upon the strengths and weaknesses prevalent in the parents' relationship. Peter was a weak conception because of what was going on with his parents at the time.

The mother, in particular, needs to be a good model because of the direct relationship she has with the child and the relationship the father has with the child through her. When the child is in her womb, it is good for the mother to have a positive outlook toward the father, the male energy, as well as a good feeling about herself as a woman. The mother needs to create a visual consciousness in her mind at this time and think of good, strong men and beautiful, healthy women. This positivity will help her child develop these same traits.

Meditating during this time is also very beneficial. When a new life is growing in the womb, nature has imbued the mother with a greater amount of soul energy. The light and love is purer. That purity is what attracts us to babies. Their soul essence is untarnished. Their light is brighter because they have just come from the other side.

Because the energy inside the womb has been increased, an elimination immediately starts to happen. That shining soul begins to push out all the toxins that have accumulated in the mother's body. This elimination is natural, especially for women who have not experienced a great deal of cleansing in their lives. If a woman's energy has not been moving in her body, the pregnancy will precipitate a greater purification when the increased vibration of energy pushes out the toxins. She will then experience "morning sickness." The vomiting loosens up the diaphragm and allows more room for the growing fetus.

When we understand that the child is a glowing soul and has a lot more energy than we do, then we can accept the responsibility of being conscious with the being that is

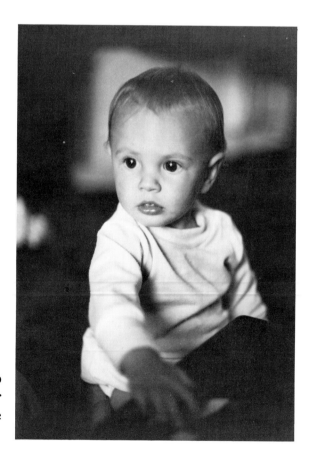

"That is what attracts us to babies...their light is brighter because they have just come from the other side."

growing inside the mother. On an energy level the baby understands everything that is happening from the time of conception onwards.

A mother's awareness work with the baby inside her is the truest indication of the baby's consciousness during pregnancy. A beautiful example of the baby's consciousness is seen during the Awareness Counseling work that we do (see Glossary). The parent talks to the fetus, the developing child. A question that often comes up is whether it is good to have sex during the pregnancy. Over and over again the child gives the same answer. "I really don't want you pounding on me a lot. It doesn't feel very comfortable. At the same time I want you to have a fulfilling husband and wife relationship. Ideally, I would like you to be celibate during this time. I have a pretty good idea that you're not able to do this, so satisfy each other so you can feel good about being together. Be creative with your sexual energy. Just keep my situation in mind and don't pound on me."

During pregnancy the whole emotional part of a woman's life, which centers in the pelvis, undergoes a tremendous change. The tightness of her emotions totally loosens up. The whole water basin, as we call the pelvis, opens up and prepares for the child to come out. When the woman finally arrives at the point of birthing, she becomes complete.

As the child pushes its way into the world, the mother is giving forth all her creative energy which, at this moment, is physically the most similar to the man's energy it will ever be for a woman. The final push of the baby is like the man's ejaculation. The child literally explodes into the world. The whole lower end of the woman totally opens up and explodes with almost superhuman force. The woman knows for the first time exactly what the male energy is all about. Before that, she had no real understanding of it other than that she would like to have it. It is her way of knowing the physical aspect of the male energy inside herself. Then she is total and complete.

At the moment of birth, the child emerges from baking in the heat of the womb. Instead of being totally attached to the body, the soul now hovers and goes in and out for another three months. "Sudden Infant Death Syndrome" may be an example of how tentatively attached the soul is to the body during this three-month period. The soul finishes its body-mind development as it proceeds through the first three months of the child's life. The full twelve-month cycle of the zodiac, which began at conception, is completed. At the end of this twelve-month cycle, the soul is literally forced to remain in the new body.

This twelve-month cycle is crucial for children who are entering a family that is unstable, insecure, and unhappy with one another. The world does not look so pleasing to these souls. What happens is that these souls hover and wait until the twelfth month (the third month after birth) when they have to decide whether to leave or to stay. These souls tend to have more "psychic energy" because during this time they see that there is more than just physical energy. These souls have a stronger association and attachment to the mental and spiritual realms, almost to the exclusion of this world, than do souls who are welcomed here with open arms and hearts. So, until the twelfth month after conception, the soul's attachment to the body is tenuous. After the twelfth month, there is finally a real being grounded in this world totally relating to the parents.

A good example of how a soul comes into the body, attaching to positive parents, is Marie, one of the children in the Fellowship. Ryan and Susan, her parents, did not think they were going to be able to have a child. They had been married eight years before coming here, and during the last three of those years they did not use any contraception although they were not actively trying to conceive. Once Ryan and Susan joined the Fellowship, they both worked very hard on themselves. They worked on their relationship in order to create fertile ground for a child to come in and grow. They developed an attitude of acceptance and appreciation for an incoming child and avoided the engulfing physical attachment many parents have. Finally, after a long time, Marie came. Marie is a Taurus: very loving, very stable, and very earthbound. She accepts what it means to be in the world. For her there is no difference between this world and the spiritual or mental realms.

Now it is interesting that when a child is born, it is often the first time someone comes between the mother and the father. A common problem for parents at this time is that the father becomes jealous of the child. This jealousy is perfectly natural. While the mother is breast-feeding the child, giving all her attention to the child, she is experiencing her sexual energy. Ask any woman who is breastfeeding and she will tell you how "peaceful" she feels when she feeds. It is the same feeling that occurs after orgasm. That sensuality is what nature gives the mother in order for her to breastfeed. So the man picks up on that energy, he senses that feeling of completion, and he gets jealous. This puts him through emotional reactions unless his intimacy and sexual relationship with his wife are satisfying. If they have that peace in their lives already, this time period will not be as traumatic.

From the twelfth month after conception when the development of our body-mind is complete to about the age of five is a period of exploration, of motor and sensory development. The male energy is the motor, the outgoing energy. The female energy is the sensory side, the receptive energy. As the child grows and develops in mind and body, the soul quality, which is very high at birth, diminishes. The more body and mind we have, the less pure soul energy shows through. In the child this soul quality manifests as innocence. As we create actions in our lives that reflect previous actions from other lives, these mental and physical impressions crystallize and move us further and further away from our connection to our soul quality. Until that time, innocence prevails.

This innocence is the reason some children, up to the ages of six or seven, are still capable of having visions and an easy relationship with God. These children can still see the light, spin out into the universe at will, and see or feel angels and elves, fairies and spirits. As we get older, these associations disappear unless we are lucky enough to have a major spiritual experience that reminds us.

Then, at the age of thirteen or so, all the sexual energy that has been dormant since the time it was used to bring us into the world bursts forth and we become young adults. Suddenly we have sexual feelings and longings and we do not know where they have come from or what to do with them. The problem in our society is that the time period when all this is happening, from approximately grades six to nine (ages eleven to fourteen), is a time of total confusion and anxiety for most young people. For them there is a huge amount of watery sexual energy, a strong pull and attraction to the opposite sex, and no way to channel it.

By providing our young adults with a positive outlet for their sexual energy, we can give them the responsibility to use this creative energy in a mature way. The purpose of this energy is for creating a child. If we do not give our children any responsibility as they become young adults, they have no way to positively direct their sexual energy. Then they end up having tremendous pain and emotional disturbances.

By the time our children reach high school, they have a totally mixed-up understanding of sex and we blame them because they lack a sense of responsibility. In fact, we as a culture encourage this lack of responsibility by treating our young adults like infants. We confuse them by giving them double messages. First we tell them to buckle down to work so they can get into college, and then they can relax. Then we tell them to have a great time in high school, because in college they will really have to buckle down to work and be responsible. Then we modify that and tell them when they are in college they will not really be adults until they have a job and earn their own livelihood. Actually, we don't know what to do with them, so our own uncertainty leads to generations of scattered, confused, and often helpless people.

The key here is to give responsibility to young adults within the home, the family, and the community. People at this age really like to feel needed and responsible. By having things to do, young people feel like the adults they really are. Responsibilities give them an outlet for the potentially overwhelming creative power that, when unleashed, can frustrate them if it is not channeled appropriately.

When the energy is in balance and we designate responsibility to our children, they become responsible adults. They will be able to willingly accept the duties that will enable them to live positively in the world. This lesson has always been the underlying motive for lemonade stands, grass mowing, and babysitting, to name a few

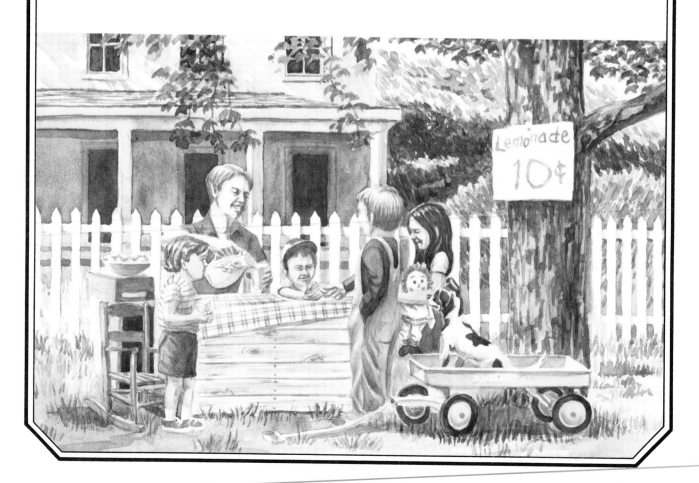

teenage jobs. What really creates a balance is for young people to contribute the money made from such jobs directly to the family. It is their way of participating in the workings of the whole family and it helps them to feel they are doing their part.

This issue of responsibility makes me think of my daughter, Liza. When Liza turned thirteen she provisionally came on staff at the Alive Fellowship for one year. Similarly, in certain religions, like Judaism for example, the child becomes an adult at thirteen and is initiated into the religious community. Liza participated in all the duties of a staff member and she was treated as one. Happily, she even contributed all her babysitting earnings to the Fellowship. This responsibility totally switched her sexual energy, which before was very confused. She was accepted as an adult, which helped her accept herself as one, too. She became very happy. Her sexual energy was being used positively, as creative energy going outward to other people to help them. In this way she helped herself. When Liza turned fourteen, after the one-year trial period, she chose to become a permanent member of the Alive Fellowship.

Towards the ages of sixteen and seventeen our sexual energy and our desire to take on responsibility reaches its peak. For centuries, in societies all over the world, this has been recognized as the appropriate time for marriage. If encouraged, people are ready for it at this age. Once again, if we discourage marriage at this age, we create infantilism in our children.

This age is really the right time to focus with one partner. We all have experienced the joy and vitality of our first love. The true feeling of commitment is really there. It is wonderful if at this time we have total support from our parents and family for taking the step of marriage. It is the best time to come together for birthing and parenting, as well. We have more vitality and youthful enthusiasm. All the energy is right there at the surface.

The ideal situation would be for both the young adults and the parents to take responsibility for finding an appropriate marriage partner. If this was done in our society, we would create a stronger base for marriages and a greater commitment to making them work. The entire family would be focusing on marriage at a time period when the vitality in young adults is present for being married and having children.

There are two ways to create this situation. The first alternative requires the young adult to take responsibility for his or her desires at this age and share those feelings with the parents. Then the parents go out and hunt for a suitable man or woman for their son or daughter. The parents might even work it out astrologically to get just the right combination for the "perfect" match. The two meet, spend some time together, and get to know one another. We used to call it courting. Then the young people can decide if it feels right or not. Either they say, "No, dad and mom, we do not feel the magic we are supposed to feel. Can we find someone else?" or they say, "Great! Can we get married?"

After going through this process, there can be no recriminations on the parents' part if the marriage does not work out. There will not be a "should" or an "I-told-you-so" about whom the child married. This family alliance would be a big switch in the United States. Everybody would have a say in the choice and a sense of responsibility in the match.

The second alternative would be for the parents to have a voice in a so-called "love marriage." It *is* possible for people to meet their knight or princess. That kind of match is valid, too. Ideally, in this situation, the children would then consult with the parents and everybody would take on joint responsibility for evaluating the potential partnership. Everyone, of course, would need to agree on this ideal and to respect one another's opinion. Let's not forget we are talking about ideals now, which means we are taking for granted that there is a high level of consciousness and receptivity on everyone's part.

Respect for our children allows them to grow up and be adults. In our society we do not let women be women until about twenty-five and men be men until about thirty. What this proposed arrangement will do is allow a whole generation of people to live more harmoniously. It will encourage young adults to go with the feelings they have at this early age period and direct those feelings in an upward spiral. Then we will be able to regenerate the family and have strong marriages which will create strong children.

Moving on to the cycle between twenty and forty years, we arrive at a time for testing out life. We still have our vitality, so it is a good time for making mistakes, finding out what works for us, and learning how to create good situations for ourselves. My father always said, "Burn your hand, Jeff, but don't burn it twice." He meant: make mistakes but don't repeat the same ones over and over. Even better, learn from the mistakes of other people so you will not have to burn your own hand at all.

This time period, from twenty to forty, is when we recognize our youth, realize our creativity, and go out into the world and gamble. Lose or win, it does not really matter, as long as we can use the understanding we gain to help us become more conscious. Life could end tomorrow so we might as well live it fully. If we hold ourselves back and retire at the age of thirty, like so many people are doing now, we will miss the lessons of this cycle of life.

For example, many young couples feel stuck and frustrated living in the city. So they create a polarity by thinking that living in the country will solve all their problems. Then they move to the country and build their dream house in the woods, plant a garden, and their minds go wild. They really start talking and listening to each other, but the same battling comes up as it did before. Their fantasy is shattered. They split up because they do not have the understanding to work through the negativity that surfaces.

I don't mean that we can't be creative and make our dreams come true. If our energy is in gardening, then we can create more energy and growth. Instead of five acres, we can farm one hundred acres. This time period is not a time for isolation and selfishness. It is a period of putting out creative energy to our nuclear family and to the human family as well. After we have been creative and taken responsibility for our creations, we can begin to relax and ease up.

When we reach anywhere from forty-five to sixty-five,

we are worldly and wise. As grandparents in this time period, we can start to let our children carry the heavier burdens of responsibility. This is the time our children can come to us for counsel and advice. In our unbalanced society this usually is not done. In America it is unfortunate that we do not feel respect for our elders. We need to develop respect for their wisdom. We send our old people to convalescent homes and put them out to pasture. We see them once in a while, if we are lucky, and usually there is something else we would rather be doing. We are unwilling to relate to our own people. We don't want to hear their feelings or nurse them in their physical and emotional pain. This lack of communication is a reflection of our own disease.

It is good for us to care for our elders as they cared for us when we were children. Old age is their time of need. It is obvious how old people become like little children, especially when they are not well. Taking care of each other is how we learn from one another. This kind of

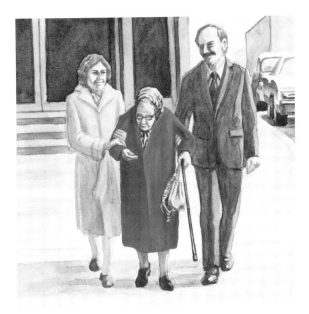

experiential learning is what being a human being is all about. As we travel through our rites of passage with consciousness, we see more and more that everyone in our life can be our teacher if we cultivate the eyes to see and the ears to hear.

My dad lived during the Depression. I have so much love and respect for my father's wisdom about the world that I naturally went to him for advice about the recession that is predicted. Everything we have been doing, like gathering food and making sure that all our payments are made, are things he suggested. He said to be sure I had food for a few months so if there was a major contraction in this country, we could all function for at least a six-month period.

Then I joked with him and asked, "Dad, do you have your food together?" He laughed and said, "No, son, you've got it!" I was so happy because he rarely shares anything like that. He was giving me his respect and trust. He was handing over to me the responsibility of taking care of him and my mother when the crunch comes. He's a meat and potatoes man and he knows the Fellowship is pure vegetarian. Yet, the bottom line for him was, "With you, Jeff, I can eat vegetables."

Finally, we arrive at the last period of transformation in our lives, our preparation for death and union with God. Ideally, our family circumstances will provide us with a sense of security and a bonding that allows us to do this work. We will be totally cared for by our sons and daughters, which does not necessarily mean we all live on the same piece of property. The bonding can be an emotional one like the one I have with my father, or it can be a practical one, if need be. Either way, it is an opportunity to come to grips with our life and our death.

Life is really elusive. First we are here and then we are gone. We come into this world and we really don't understand how or why. We live our allotted amount of time and then we leave this world. The thing to understand about death is that it is another part of life. We come into this world with pain and we leave this world with pain. How much pain we have when we die depends on how much work we have done on ourselves during our lives and how much preparation we have made.

If we totally negate death and refuse to look at it, then we have no understanding of what life encompasses. Death will be a very painful experience because we have not accepted the part it plays as the highest time of our life. Just as birth is a reaction, so is death. Reaction creates pain and reaction is emotional. The less emotional we are, the more conscious we can be and the less pain we will experience. That goes for life as well as death. The formula for life and death is the same.

So, the more conscious we are, the less emotion and the less pain we will have in life as well as in death. Then we can smile at death. The more emotional we are, the less conscious we will be and the greater pain we will have when we die. We will be resisting and reacting rather than accepting death and being conscious during the ultimate experience of life.

As we get older, it is much easier for us to consciously leave our body and then consciously come back into the world. Going and coming is as easy for old people as it is for babies. When everything is functioning well for us as old people, it is easy to make the transition back and forth. Birth and death are simply ways to learn how to be conscious in the human body-mind, coming into and going out of this world. Life is learning how to be conscious in either direction. Once we learn how to come in consciously, be here consciously, and go out consciously, we will truly understand that there is no death. There is only a transformation in consciousness.

VII

Marriage:
A Commitment to Growth

Marriage itself, as an institution, is one of the best forms we have for bringing about healing in people. The reason for this is that in marriage we have a man and a woman who focus their attention on each other and allow themselves to come close to each other. When they focus on each other and bring their concentration and their feelings toward each other, then they have a wonderful opportunity to step on each other's toes, to create a lot of pain, a lot of disharmony, and a lot of argument. All of these things provide wonderful opportunities for growth.

Marriage is a form that brings people together to focus their entire maleness and femaleness with each other. I have been married six years now and I have learned a great deal. Sharon, my wife, likes to call marriage a life-long healing crisis. I feel this description is appropriate when we understand exactly what a healing crisis entails.

A healing crisis is a situation which occurs when a person's soul energy increases within their body-mind and becomes stronger than their lower mind. The increased energy comes from a heightened awareness at the mental, physical, and emotional levels. When the soul vibration is bigger than the physical body, the higher mind is influenced by the soul. Then we experience symptoms of disease as part of the healing process. Automatically, the body, the mind, and the spirit push out the toxins of past associations, past relationships, and past diseases; an elimination takes place at all levels. This healing is exactly what marriage encourages.

For a man, the woman he marries is an externalization of his inner woman. For a woman, the man she marries is a reflection of her male energy. When you see Sharon, my wife, you are looking at my vision of a woman. In other words, she embodies the qualities I am attracted to in a woman. In a physical form, Sharon is a slower, denser vibration of my feminine side.

This understanding, for both men and women, means that marriage definitely becomes a healing crisis because we are constantly dealing with that part of ourselves on the outside that we most likely do not like to deal with on the inside. Marriage forces us to confront ourselves, and as a result our consciousness grows. We are both attracted and repelled by the polarity inside ourselves. So when we can come to the acceptance of our marriage partner we can come to the acceptance of ourselves. That means when I accept Sharon's femininity, I accept my own feminine side.

A man marries his mother, and a woman marries her

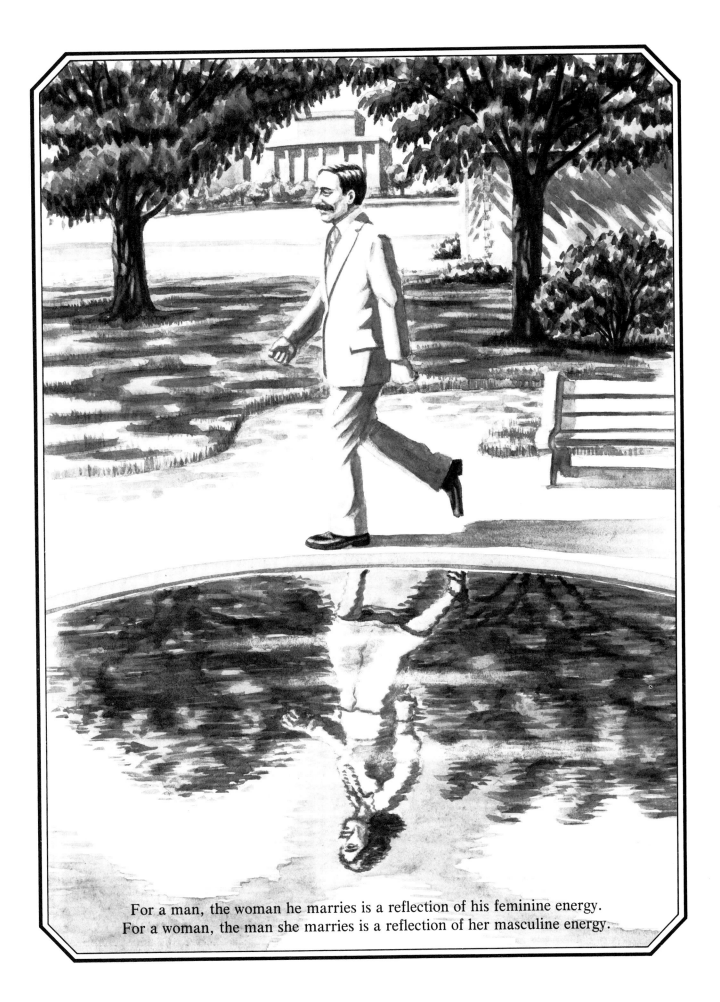

For a man, the woman he marries is a reflection of his feminine energy.
For a woman, the man she marries is a reflection of her masculine energy.

father. Men learn the qualities of feminine energy from their mothers. So they marry women who are reflections of the mother inside themselves. Each one of us is made up physically, mentally, and emotionally of our father and our mother. So for a man, his wife reflects his mother (his first woman), Mother Nature, Mother Earth, the Universal Mother. Furthermore, the woman or man we are attracted to for a marriage partner will naturally have very much the same emotional make-up, the same emotional work, the same buttons to press, as we do. Our partner will be a reflection of our secondary energy.

My wife, Sharon, for instance, is a very powerful woman. She is really beautiful and there is a lot of her. Sharon is also very nurturing and she gives a lot of service. She is strong-willed, domineering, and sometimes stubborn. Now that is all a reflection of my feminine energy. I mean, if you were to describe me, you could use those very words. I am stubborn, strong-willed, domineering, powerful, receptive, I give service, and there is a lot of me.

I think marriage is one of the most misunderstood institutions in our country. We have no real training, no education, for people who want to be married. There is a lack of focus on the realities of married life. There is no forum for expressing feelings about what it is like to be married, the pitfalls to look out for, or the hazards that will need to be surmounted. So when the difficulties of marriage arise, nobody has been forewarned. Then most people say, "Oh, this is my unique situation. I am the only one who goes through things like this." Then, immediately, the desire to separate enters the mind and we usually act upon that desire. Instead of reacting to our negative desires, we need to understand that in married life we are going to feel negative things about the person we are with. It is totally impossible not to.

We think we are going to be in the courting stage of the relationship for our whole life. We live in this fantasy and never really come to the point of accepting what marriage is all about. Courting is not marriage. Courting is the first stage of a relationship. It is when we show all of our positivity to the other person; when we put on our best dress, our best suit, our best manners, and the most acceptable feelings and emotions we can muster in order to attract the other person. The courting stage is when we sell ourselves.

Marriage is literally buying something. We all know that whenever we buy something, it does not always turn out to be quite what we thought it was when we finally get it home. When we buy something, we have the responsibility of taking care of it. In that respect marriage is also very much like a plant. Both need good fertile soil in order to grow. We get that fertile soil from the work we do on ourselves before we get married.

Most marriages start out as an emotional relationship rather than a spiritual relationship. This emotional beginning is the reason there is so much disappointment and confusion when the emotional attraction wears off. The emotional attraction we feel initially is a reaction. We immediately react at an emotional, unconscious level to the other person. Suddenly, there is this incredible feeling and we think, "Oh, I'm so attracted, Woweee!" Then we proclaim this attraction as our inner feeling: our soul has found its mate. In fact, this emotional attraction, this feeling, is actually sexual attraction. It is unconscious and does not last.

True love means not being attached to each other's negativity in any way. When we are truly loving each other, each person has the freedom for their soul quality, which is inside, to manifest outside. The soul quality takes a long time to come out. Nurturing each other's soul quality takes understanding and patience from both partners. When we give this nurturing to each other from a place of love and devotion, the soul quality becomes stronger than the mind. Most of us expect our soul qualities to manifest from the lower part of ourselves, the unconscious, emotional part rather than from the higher, conscious part of ourselves.

When we relate with deep feeling at a high level of consciousness with another person, there will be no problem five or six years later with a statement like, "I married this person? This isn't the person I married." Anytime I hear this statement I know they married the other person emotionally and not consciously. Their attraction was an emotional reaction and not from the realm of the higher mind.

So the first step in marriage is to understand what it is all about and recognize its power. What I'm saying is, "Recognize the power of polarity, of putting a man and a woman together for the rest of their lives and understand that it means making a commitment for the rest of our lives to marriage itself." The commitment is to marry marriage.

If we marry like most people do (I would say like

ninety-five percent of the people who marry today), we marry out of love, and that love is emotional and unconscious, with no real depth of feeling and no real awareness about who the other person really is. Then we set ourselves up for a great fall. I mean, let's face it. We often become disillusioned when we get close to someone.

Disillusionment brings up another emotion that affects a marriage greatly and that emotion is hate. About ninety-five per cent of us sometimes hate ourselves deeply. When we feel that hatred in ourselves it has to follow that we will also hate the person that is right there in front of us. When the hatred comes up, the mind goes even further and says, "If I hate this person, then we shouldn't stay married." This mental pattern is the reason there are so many failed marriages today. Every time one person starts to feel that hate in themselves, and then for the other person as well, the marriage immediately ends and there is the pain of separation and divorce.

Due to this separation and divorce, the power of having children is lost. I mean right now, today, about one out of every two children that comes into the world in America is going to have to have a separated mother and father. These children will not have the benefit of both parents living together with them. The high rate of divorce in this country is an imbalance that needs attention and real focus.

When we quickly and thoughtlessly divorce, we teach our children how to be selfish. We actually perpetuate our own selfishness by passing it on to our children. Approximately half of the children in this country today are going to be selfish, really selfish, because they have learned that quality from their mothers and fathers. These children know that their mothers and fathers are very selfish because they feel the lack of commitment and responsibility their parents showed towards bearing and raising them.

Now, children of divorced parents are more likely to be selfish in their own marriages. I see it all the time with students in the Alive Polarity programs. The disease patterns of the parents are passed on to their children. Therefore, children of divorced parents, and people who themselves have been divorced, know what work they need to do in their lives. They need to work on their commitment to marriage and to understand what that commitment is all about. They need to go through all the pain and selfishness they have in themselves, or that they have experienced through their parents, and learn from that pain.

When I talk about working on the commitment to marriage, I mean working on the commitment to growth. In marriage we grow beyond ourselves because marriage is beyond the self. In other words, when we are truly married, it is totally impossible to be selfish anymore. Marriage is the death of the single ego. In a good marriage we think about the other person before we think about ourselves. Marriage is all about giving and forgiving, it is about serving the other person and putting him or her first. That service is the power in marriage.

At the marriage ceremony, we stand up in front of everyone and make a commitment to the other person and to the world that we are together as a couple. We are committing ourselves to being with this other person. And "being with" means helping the other person by giving ourselves to them. So by being committed to marriage, we commit ourselves to staying with the other person "for better or worse, in sickness and in health." That commitment means we can go through the hate when it comes up without leaving or even threatening to leave.

We will all go through that time of hatred. I have not known anyone who has been married who has not hated the other person sometime during their marriage. Hate is an unconscious emotional reaction which we all have. In marriage, hate will be stirred up and brought to the surface.

The power of the positivity, the concentration, and the love that is focused on another person in a marriage automatically brings up a healing crisis. All that positivity and focus squeezes out the negativity of the past. The hate surfaces. Marriage brings up the dirt of the negative mind.

So by having our commitment to marriage and not to the other person, we come closer to our partner than ever before. Instead of hating the other person, instead of rejecting them, moving away, withdrawing, closing off, and separating, we go through the hate. Then, in this world of polarity, a wonderful thing happens. On the other side of the hate is great emotional attachment, which we call love. We know that our love is going to have to come, because if we hate that much, we also have that much love and attachment. It's the old story: when we get into a big fight, making up later is all the more fun. This cycle always happens that way.

So by having the commitment to marriage, we will go

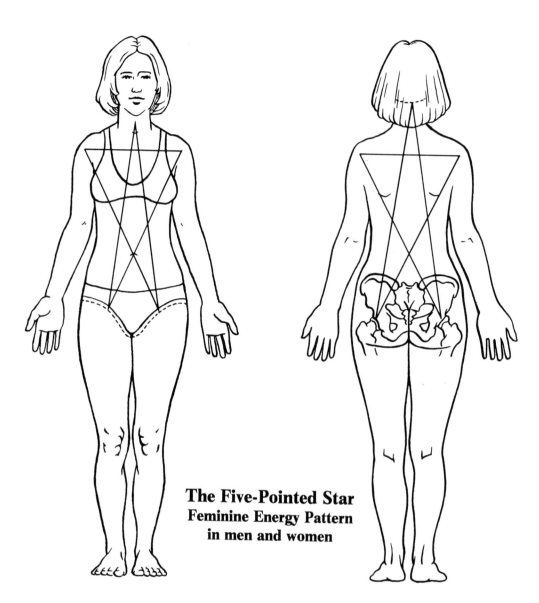

The Five-Pointed Star
Feminine Energy Pattern
in men and women

The five and six-pointed stars are practical tools for visualizing imbalances in the male and female energies of each individual. Any imbalances along these lines of energy reflect the mental, emotional and physical patterns that create disease. Imbalances can be seen physically as high or low shoulders, raised or lowered hips, tipped sacrums, and constricted or expanded pelvises or chests, to name a few indications.

Heart diseases, back, and spine problems may be a result of imbalances in the six-pointed star: the masculine, outgoing, motor energy or fire principle in the body. Cancer may be caused by an imbalance in the five-pointed star: the feminine, receptive, sensory energy or water principle in the body.

Within the deep commitment of marriage, we can develop balanced family

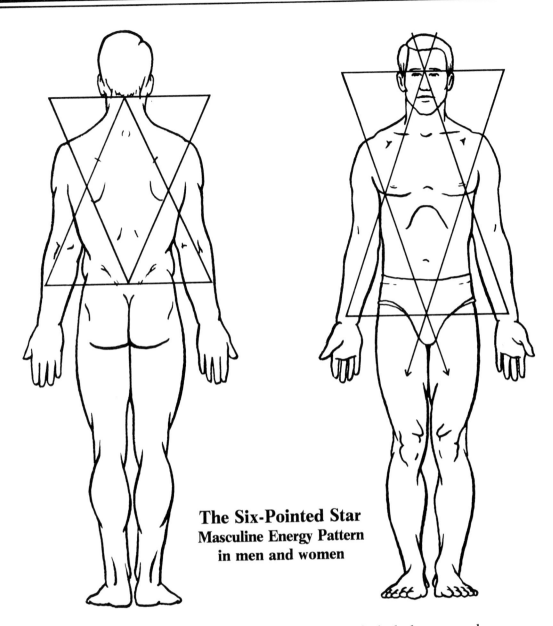

The Six-Pointed Star
Masculine Energy Pattern
in men and women

relationships by doing the emotional work that heals chronic imbalances and prevents disease. In a committed marriage, the process of continual reflection between the man and the woman creates an environment that encourages positive growth and harmonious living.

When we are unmarried, by remaining celibate and focusing our energy on our relationship with God, we can also create a healing situation. Through our focus, God can work with us, manifesting our complementary energy, and serve as a reflection in the same way as a husband or wife. With the sincere commitment to working on ourselves, we can be celibate, love the Lord, and still be balanced. This understanding is the essence of what it means to be a nun or a priest, in any religion, and be married to God.

through the hate and through the elimination of negative emotions that are brought up to the surface. They will then be squeezed out. Our commitment to marriage will bring us through the unconscious emotional reactions that usually send couples running for a divorce. Every time we go through all that hate and reach the other side, God, working through nature, gives us more understanding. We let go of our immaturity and become more mature, less selfish, and less self-oriented. We then develop the quality of compassion towards our fellow human beings.

What I am saying is very simple. We have to concentrate our energy and make our commitment to marriage and not to the other person. Then we will accept marriage and the commitment we have made to focus all our attention, including our sexual energy, on one person for the rest of our lives.

For me, my wife Sharon is all the women in the world. Now that is a lot of focus. That focus also means a lot of power. In order for us to have this kind of focus, we need to have a commitment to a form that can bring about a marriage relationship capable of handling that much power and that much love. The love I am talking about is spiritual love, love for God, love for something that is more than ourselves.

The commitment in marriage is to a positive attachment, a commitment to be devoted to something beyond both partners. This kind of love is the only kind of love that will create a strong foundation for a marriage. An emotional attraction fades quickly. Without a spiritual commitment to the God in the other person, to the soul quality in the other person, there is no chance of weathering the storms that will arise.

Today we are selfish. We usually only think of ourselves. If we do not get something our own way, if we do not get touched in just the right place, if we do not get what we feel we need in a marriage, we immediately look for another relationship that will provide us with what we want. We search for that "perfect" situation in which we will "live happily ever after." What I want to share with you is that there is no such relationship. We can keep on changing marriage partners and our work with each one will always be the same. We will always marry our work.

The only way to transcend the problems that come up in a marriage is to commit ourselves to that marriage in the same state of mind we commit ourselves to having children. When a child is born it has a mother and a father for the rest of its life. That interrelationship is there and cannot be broken. The same sense of commitment and responsibility has to be present when going into a marriage. We need to marry as if we are having children. Marriage needs the same focus. It is the same lifelong commitment and we must recognize that.

Most people enter marriages today with thoughts like, "Oh, I'll marry for five or ten years and if it lasts that long then I'll decide if I'm going to have children. If we don't get along, we can always get a divorce." With this attitude, we cannot have a marriage. That is really just living together. It is not what marriage is all about.

What I am saying is that when we are parents, we are committed to, and responsible for, our children for the rest of our lives. If we do not take that responsibility, we are not being a parent; we are not being a mother or a father. Marriage needs the same focus as having children. Marriage is the same life-long commitment. So I suggest, if you are planning to get married, think about it in terms of having children, whether you are having children or not. If you cannot make that type of commitment, then do not get married. Marriage is not for you.

If marriage is not for you, be with yourself and be self-oriented. That's okay too, as long as you work on yourself. Working on yourself will bring you closer to God, closer to something higher than yourself. I want to tell you, no matter what you do in this life, you are going to want and need something more than yourself. Being a human being is not just about the self.

So, if you want to have children, then get married. And if you want to live with someone for the rest of your life, marry them as if you want to have children with them. It does not necessarily mean you must have children. What it does mean is that you must take the attitude that you are going to have children and you will have a connection with that person for the rest of your life. That responsibility is the essence of the commitment.

Some of the most emotional situations we have today, as modern Americans and modern Westerners, have to do with security and insecurity. It is really clear to me that the insecurity that has developed within our society in the last fifty years comes from the erosion of the institution of marriage. Marriage in America has lost its importance and its value.

What has followed from the situation of marriage losing its value is that all of our commitments have broken down. In our commitments to other people, other relationships, our work, in virtually all aspects of our lives, we are seeing the disintegration of the value of a contract. These days it is almost useless to sign a contract with another person because the likelihood that it will be broken is almost a certainty.

In terms of human relationships, marriage is the most solid contract that we can make. When we can be committed and responsible within a marriage, our commitments to ourselves, to our children, to our work, and to our fellow human beings will be solid. Our word, which is a sign of integrity here in the West, will then be worth something. Our word will be valued. So being married and using the power of marriage brings value, worth, and commitment to our ideals. Those ideals become valuable because they are backed by sincere devotion to service; serving something, or someone, beyond ourselves.

What it all comes down to is concentrating our energy instead of scattering it. It is perfectly natural to have sexual energy, and it is part of being human to want to attach to other people. So we might as well use those challenges as opportunities to practice positive attachment and focus that energy on another human being with a deep sense of commitment and loyalty.

When we are capable of developing a deep inner relationship with our partner in marriage, it will follow naturally that we will be able to do the same thing with our fellow human beings. Responsible marriages encourage the sense of community within our society that is lacking today. This lack of a deeper sense of community has led to an escalation of fear and insecurity throughout our whole country. The marriage commitment is a form from which we can draw the power to stabilize and re-build the fabric of our crumbling society.

VIII

Parenting:
We are All Parents and We are All Children

The main thing to understand about being a parent is that we become a parent whenever we are with children. It does not matter whether we are their blood parents or not. Anyone who works with children is a parent because parents are examples. When we are in the position of being an example to children, we are being watched. Both the good things and the bad things we do are copied and imitated. We are all parents and we are all teachers. It is part of being human.

The core of the psychological work we do at the Alive Fellowship is parenting. It is the real teaching. Some people think the work we are doing is "esoteric" or "new age." Actually, all esoteric teaching really consists of is learning how to deal with a strong mind. The real work we do involves getting into feelings and emotions and understanding the mind. This work is very simple because the truth is very simple. As we learn about ourselves and who we are, we learn what parenting is all about.

Once we take responsibility for being a parent-teacher, it is essential to understand one fact: we will all make mistakes. Wisdom comes from the understanding that once we make a mistake we need to learn from it and not repeat the same mistake again. Then our children will learn that it is alright to make mistakes. They will learn from their mistakes and not repeat them again and again.

Learning from mistakes is human and a wonderful quality to pass on to children. By our example we can teach children how to be human. When we are being an example, we are taking responsibility to be the best person we can possibly be. We are accepting the grace that we have been given as parents and we are passing that grace on to our children.

All mothers and fathers, no matter who they are or what they do, truly want the best for their children. It is one of the "always" statements we can say about the world and there are not too many of those. In order to give our best to children, we need to determine for ourselves what will make us the best human beings we can possibly be. When we pass that experience on to our children, they will be able to learn what it is to be good human beings in their own right.

Our real job, then, is first to understand what it means to be a child. Children are human beings consisting of light and energy. They are people who know everything we are thinking, saying, and feeling and know it even from the time of conception. Everything an expectant mother eats, thinks, says, feels, and does goes directly into the child she is carrying in her womb. We can never get as close to another human being as a mother can when she is carrying a child. We can even start communicating to children when they are in the womb when we understand and accept that the child thinks in the same way we do.

When a husband and wife work together with the child from the time it is in the womb, they can reverse entire negative life patterns and transform the negative relationships between themselves and the incoming child into healing ones. This is a wonderful, powerful time when a mother can literally change her life, her life with her husband, and the life of the child she is bearing by using all of her positivity and concentration to literally court the child. That means getting to know the child and letting the child know her.

At the Alive Fellowship we do Awareness Counseling (see Glossary), which is a great way to work on our emotions. I have facilitated many, many awarenesses with children in the womb. Anytime I see parents that are being negative, and the mother has a child in her womb, I tell the mother to put the child in the chair. When the mother switches over and becomes the baby, the baby is totally clear. In the awareness the baby says exactly what the mother needs to hear and do; whatever the baby says is truthful, sincere, and conscious. Through the awareness, the child really straightens out the parents; then the parents cry and say they are sorry and the family automatically becomes closer, stronger, and more aware of each other. So the power to switch comes from the child within the womb. The child is a vibration, a new soul, a consciousness coming from a higher and finer vibration than our own. It is imperative that we, as parents, tune into the clarity that comes from the child's vibration and what that soul can teach us.

It is revolutionary for us to understand that children are people who think just as we do. Children pick up the energy of everything that is happening even though they do not literally understand our words. In fact, they are more receptive to our communication when they are in the womb and during the first year than they are later on because during that time they are still in the ether. The ether is the quality of discrimination and it is found in the throat, at the center of our emotions. When the child is in the womb it is in the ether where the emotional body is being developed and hardened by the same heat that creates the bones, the blood vessels, and the rest of the body.

Our emotional qualities, our way of being in the world and how we react to the world, are learned during the time we are in the womb until the time of birth. Because of our sexual attachment to our mother, we take on her emotional reactions. We take on our father's emotions through our mother's reactions to him. At birth our emotions are activated by the breath and projected out into the world. As we begin the detachment process and start to project ourselves as independent sexual beings, we have our own learned emotions and sexual patterns which have all been conveyed to us through our direct sexual attachment to our mother.

Some people think that when the child is in the womb it is having a wonderful experience. They think that the child is lying in there having a gay old time. Not at all. It's hell in there. The child is in an oven. It is right next to the solar plexus where the mother's fire center is located. It is really hot in there because that heat is what is used to form the child's bones.

Originally the fetus forms from the union of a sperm and an egg. The fetus is watery in its center. In order to create the alchemy of transmuting the water into earth, we need the fire which is heat. So it is very hot inside the womb while the child is being baked. The child is going through a great deal of pain. This is not a joyous time for the child. It is crying out and asking for help from the Lord. When the child comes out, it is really relieved to be out of that inferno. This is one reason that children, after a birth, seem so happy to see us. They are really happy to get out of the hell in there.

For a child who has gone through a difficult birth or, for example, if the child is not wanted, the child's soul and mind can leave the body and hover away from it for up to three months after birth. When the full twelve-month cycle of the zodiac is complete, the soul and mind have to choose whether or not to be totally in the body.

People who have gone through a traumatic birth will be more aware of the astral and emotional parts of their minds. These people develop a stronger and clearer relationship with the lighter, more sensitive, astral part of themselves. Now that does not mean the astral is more fantastic than the physical, it just means that these people have more of an awareness of it. Actually, the astral is just a trap, maybe even more of a trap than the physical mind and emotions.

So what I want to share with you is that children are people who are happy to be with us. They have found themselves in a situation where they can grow even though they do not yet have our capabilities. It is interesting to think that just nine months earlier, before conception, the child could have had an incarnation as a skier, going down a mountain with great coordination and skill; that soul could have had any number of different types of bodies. Now the soul has a brand new body and has to go through growing pains once again. When we can understand the child's pain, we can start to communicate with the child. We will be able to talk to the child and be with the child as a human being. We will be able to see the adult in the child.

Babies come into this world from a higher and finer vibration and they learn to be in this world through imitation of what they see around them. They do not know what this world is like. So, what do the parents usually do? When the child comes into this world, the parents mimic the baby. When the baby is attempting to talk, the parents say, "Goo, goo, ga, goo," grunting at the baby. Instead of the baby imitating the parents, it is the parents who are imitating the baby. The parents act as if the baby does not know or understand anything. They figure that since babies cannot talk, they also cannot know what is happening. What parents need to realize is that babies know everything that is being said and everything that is happening.

We treat a dog as if it knows everything we are saying and as if it understands what is going on, but we will not treat babies the same way. I often watch parents imitating their babies because they are so attached to them. They say, "Goo, goo, ga, ga, I love you." There is so much love when the words are spoken that the children trust their parents. Soon the children grow up talking baby talk until somewhere along the line the children realize that the words they learned from their parents do not have any meaning. Then they become disappointed and disillusioned when they realize that their parents have taught them nonsense.

So we end up having four year old babies, twenty-five year old babies, and even fifty and sixty year old babies who never learn or accept what it is to be an adult. When we are able to understand our effect on children, we will realize that a child is alive, a human being, an energy, a conscious soul. When we finally accept that children are conscious souls, we will communicate with them on a mature level.

Here is a story that may illustrate our misunderstanding more graphically. During the Viet Nam War, a great many men developed what is called aphasia. Aphasics go into a kind of shock in reaction to a traumatic experience. These people are not able to speak, which is a weakness in their motor ability, the male energy. At the same time, their minds are functioning like ours. I worked with some psychologists who had done experiments with aphasics. The doctors found that the aphasics were going insane only because they were being treated as insane.

When the aphasics came home from the war, what did their wives and loved ones do? They started yelling at them and mimicking them. Everyone thought the aphasics were weird because they could not communicate like everyone else. Their wives did not want to make love with them anymore or treat them normally. Soon the men became totally deranged and frustrated because there was a person inside them saying, "I'm a person. I'm alive. I'm thinking just like you're thinking." Meanwhile, everyone around them is feeling, "Ugh, he's so weird, we can't communicate with him."

One of the doctors I worked with had understood that the mind of an aphasic was normal and undamaged. He once conducted an experiment: he worked with the wife of a man who was an aphasic after the Korean War. He said, "Look, I want you to have a regular family life with your husband. I want you to go to bed with him, have sex with him, love him, and care for him just as if he was normal. Take him to visit the place where he used to work. Make everything in his life as it was previously."

So, she treated her husband normally. She kept everything out in the open and even argued with him over the things they used to argue about. The doctor who narrated this story revealed that his patient was the aphasic. He had regained his speech and emotional stability by going through this experiment with his wife.

Infants are aphasics. Their motor energy is weak and they are unable to speak, even though their minds think just like our minds think. With this awareness, we will treat our infants totally different than the way we treat them now. We wonder how our children get so mixed up. They get mixed up because we are mixed up. Luckily, the soul quality will emerge no matter what happens. In time, there will always be a solution.

The next thing to understand is that our emotional patterns are the same as our parents' emotional patterns, and we can learn from their positivity and negativity. We will not be good parents ourselves until we get clear with, and accept, the negativity and hatred we have for our own parents. We need to learn how to take the positivity from our parents and pass that on to our children.

I know for myself that it was not until I started raising children of my own that I developed an appreciation and sympathy for my own parents. When we have children of our own and we are changing their diapers, and they are screaming and peeing all over the place, we suddenly have a flash of compassion for what our parents did for us. We understand what they were going through when we were being brats and not respecting them as parents.

What we need to realize is that we come into this world purely out of attachment. So we must do the work of accepting the attachment and the closeness we have to our parents, especially to our mothers. We can never be as close to anyone as we are to our mothers.

The desire for closeness is one reason women want to have children. Women do not like to "get it on" sexually in the same way men do. Men like to penetrate. Women like to cuddle and be affectionate. Their sexual fulfillment occurs when they feel that closeness. How much closer can a woman get to another person than to have a child in her body? A mother can feel the child growing and kicking. She can feel all the child's emotions and everything else the child is going through. This closeness is the precise reason we also end up hating our mothers. When we are close to someone, we become attached to their positivity and negativity. Everybody will have some hatred in them towards their mother at some time. Of course, out of that hatred comes our love for her because we are very attached to her.

To come into the world in the first place, we need to have positive and negative attachments. We are attached to our parents through good and bad associations. Whether there is going to be more positive or negative karma depends on the individual relationship between two people. It depends on who owed what to whom. If the parents owe positive karma to the child, then the child will be receiving more good karmas. If they owe negative karma to the child, then life for the child may be very difficult.

We are attracted into this world to learn the lessons we need to learn. These lessons will become obvious from the situations that occur in our lives. The negativity we experience contains the lessons which help us grow. Once we learn the lessons, we do not have to do those negative things anymore. When our parents do negative things to us, it is important to keep in mind that we can learn from their actions. We do not have to repeat those negative patterns our parents gave us or pass them on to the next generation. So even in the midst of negativity there is positivity and an opportunity for growth.

Let's face it. The same positivity and negativity we see in our parents is in ourselves. We inherit everything. There is no such thing as a little bit here and a little bit there. When the sperm and egg meet and merge, we get it all. We get both parents' positivity and negativity. We need to move toward this realization so we can eventually learn from both parents and both sides of their personalities.

We can learn from negativity by seeing what the negativity is about and not repeating it again. Then we do not make the same mistakes twice. If we do not learn from the mistakes, the same negative patterns will repeat themselves in the next generation of children that we have. If we do not identify the patterns and reverse them, the same patterns will come up in us again and again with any person to whom we become deeply attached.

As I mentioned, we are very attached to our mother. She is the earth, the nurturing quality of Mother Nature. Since we are all on the earth, we all have the nurturing quality of a mother inside of us whether we are a man or a woman.

The way we can free ourselves from our attachment to our mother is by admitting first that we are very much attached to her. By coming to accept who our mother is, her personality, her emotional patterns, everything about her (including the part we hate), we come to accept our relationship with her. We accept that there is a purpose for which we have come together and we know that we have karma to balance with each other.

Even though we are closer to our mother, the same principle of detachment and balancing applies with our father. Men are always a little bit more aloof. Men are the heaven as defined in the *I-Ching*. Women are the earth. Right now, we are all on the earth, not in heaven. So we are going to be much closer to our mother than our father. Our father is going to stand back a bit and be an observer.

Sometimes we wish that our father was as close to us as our mother, and that is when we make a mistake. We need to learn to accept the distance that men have, that our father has, and that way we learn what it is to be the observer and see the positivity of what that distance creates. Negatively, we can also realize the mistakes that arise from creating distance and being the observer. We can learn from both sides of everything.

Learning from both the negativity and the positivity of our parents helps us to be better parents. In all the awarenesses I have seen there has never been a situation where there was total negativity or total positivity. The part to understand is that we are in this world because we have both positivity and negativity in us. Life is a school and if we were totally positive and totally perfect, we would be graduated from this school, we would not be here. If we were totally negative, we would be in a different school, one of a lower vibration.

The understanding that I am sharing about positivity and negativity means there is a combination of heaven and hell on this earth, a combination of total consciousness and total destruction. This earth is a blending of both. It's the same story with our parents. Our relationship with them will have a little bit of heaven and a little bit of hell; it will be a mixture of the two. Now it might be eighty per cent hell and twenty percent heaven or the other way around. In India they call it good karmas and bad karmas. The *I-Ching* talks about it being "the way it is," or "the way we open the book." Call it what we like, it all depends on our positivity and negativity and to which of them we decide to attach.

Every human being has both a parent and a child within them. We all remember what it is to be a child and since every child has a parent, every child also knows what it is to be a parent. The more we are able to understand this concept, the more we will recognize that adults are children and children are adults. Once we have gotten clear with our parents, we can accept the body, mind, and spirit of our baby as a reflection of ourselves, of the child inside ourselves. Then we can recognize the sameness that there is between child and adult, parent and child, mother and child, father and child, mother and son, father and son, mother and daughter, and father and daughter. The same human qualities are present in all these relationships.

We are made up of our parents' emotional patterns, and our children are made up of ours. This statement is another basic of parenting. Our children are the work we have been given to do. Everything in our children is a reflection of us, a reflection of the work we need to do in the world. We can use the astrological signs in our child's birth chart to show us this work. So, if we have a Taurus child, our work is to learn what it is to be a Taurus. The reason we all incarnate into this world together, as a family, as a group, is that we are each other's work. We actually pull our children into the creation with our attachment to their particular souls.

As I said before, our child is a reflection of the child in us. So if we are going to be conscious adults, we need to give up the immature part of ourselves, the bratty child, and keep the innocent part of ourselves which is the true child. The innocent child does not indulge in hard-core sex, lying, cheating, or anything hurtful. The innocent child is honest, sincere, and sensitive.

We need to let go of the child in ourselves that is bratty, selfish, and sensual; the one who needs to constantly touch, feel, and experience in order to be in the world. Unfortunately, we usually hold onto that part of the child in ourselves, the one who is constantly experimenting and testing. What we really need to do is hold onto the part of ourselves that is innocent, sensitive, and trusting as well as trustworthy.

This understanding of the child within us is crucial if we are going to understand our relationship to children, in whatever contact we have with them, especially if they belong to us. The work we do on ourselves directly influences the behavior of the children we parent-teach.

For example, if the parents have been really conscious and have done emotional work with the child since conception, the child will have more awareness. This conscious work on ourselves and the child pays off in easier discipline and constant re-clarification of inner work for both parents and child. When the child needs discipline in any situation, all that will be needed is a very clear, conscious statement with feeling and power in it. This statement will cause the child to switch whatever negative behavior it is exhibiting.

The beauty and power of being a parent was very obvious in an incident here at Alive Polarity involving Susan Costello and her daughter, Marie. One day, when Susan was disciplining Marie, I heard Susan say, "Marie, you're acting like a brat and you're being really selfish." Marie did not respond to this statement.

Now, in order for Susan to have this statement make an impact on Marie, Susan had to truly let go of her own negativity and let go of the brat she was with her own parents. When Susan told Marie she was acting like a brat she suddenly realized, "Oh, my God, that means I have to let go of my brat." About a half hour later, after Susan had done an awareness, she again told Marie she was acting like a selfish brat. This time there was an immediate response, and I have noticed that Marie has not been a spoiled brat to that degree since this episode.

So, what I am teaching is that there is actually an opportunity for growth in consciousness for everybody involved when a child is being a brat. Having a child is sort of like having a Saturn return. Like Saturn, the child brings up to the surface all the negativity that is deep inside us.

When we can say to a child, "Okay, I've really ended my brat and now it's time for it to end in you," then it can end. If our negative pattern does not end, then it is not going to end in our child. This is true of any negative pattern. Unless we switch our own negativity to positivity, we cannot give our statements the strength, commitment, clarity, and consciousness that is needed to switch the child. Once again, the child is simply a reflection of who we are and everything we have been up until that moment.

Instead of getting caught up in negativity, we need to learn how to attach to the positivity in the world. For example, when I make a decision, I focus on all the positivity in each of the different options connected to that particular event. We all find it a lot easier to get bogged down in negativity rather than focus on the positivity. To avoid this trap I do not concentrate on any of the negativity.

When it comes time to make my decision, I go with the option that offers the most positive possibilities because in the positivity is movement, creativity, and God. I have come to recognize these masculine qualities as the energy that gives me a direction and a form to follow. Here's a good example. Let's say our parents are eighty percent positive and one day they really blow it and beat us up. We get bruised and remember the beating for years and years. We hate them for it. That beating accounts for the twenty percent rotten part in them. What happens to most of us is that we take that twenty percent negativity and use it to negate the eighty percent positivity by carrying hatred for our parents in our hearts and minds for years.

Harboring resentment is exactly what causes disease in the body. That focus on the negative, that resentment, ferments and ferments, and we end up with cancer at thirty years old or leukemia at one year old. To avoid the disease, we need to come to the acceptance of the negativity. We need to be forgiving. Then, we can focus on the positivity and not end up negating ourselves. Now that is truly positive.

When we attach negatively to someone, we are doing it out of selfishness. In other words, "I'm acting this way to get something from you, and I know if I continue to act this way you'll give me what I want." So, if we are attached to our parents negatively, it is often because we want to stay a child with them. Childhood was a good time in our lives and we can get a certain kind of attention and reward by being a child again. Similarly, every time our parents are with us they continue to treat us like a child because that is how they remember us. It was a good time for them, too.

When we start to attach to the positivity in our parents, our parents will start treating us like another individual in the world. They will be able to accept our child-like qualities without treating us like a child. They will recognize the youth and enthusiasm that we have and they will respect those qualities in us.

Nature is a great teacher of this difficult lesson. When a bird gets kicked out of the nest, it is not that the mother is being harsh or unloving. It is just the opposite. What the mother is saying is, "You're a bird and birds fly. You've got wings and unless you use those wings they're going to get stuck to your body and you'll never fulfill your destiny to be a bird. So, out you go." The bird goes out and it has to fly because it has wings. It may flap a bit, even hit the ground and tumble along until it gets the hang of it, but it does go out and becomes fully itself.

So we see that being a parent is one of the more maturing and refining processes we can go through as human beings. By being parents we get to see, experience, and remember our own childhood. We are able to let out the child inside us and play easily with children.

If we really learn about ourselves as adults, we will be right there waiting to help children when they begin to go beyond their boundaries. Boundaries are important in parent-teaching because this world we live in is a limited world. We must have boundaries in order to live within it successfully and fully. A lake has boundaries around it so the fish can swim in it. By giving children boundaries and limitations, the day will come when the children will know how to be in the world, "how to swim in it," and they will be happy.

It is when we do not give limitations and boundaries

that children get confused and grow up not knowing how to be adults. Children then lose their relationship to the world and start to destroy themselves. This confusion is one of the reasons we have so many suicides in our society. People do not know, or have not learned, their limitations.

We need to show children what their limitations are. As their limitations broaden, children become more conscious. As children grow, we can make the boundaries bigger and bigger, until finally, when children become adults, their boundary is the whole earth.

So, the next basic of parenting is to give children form, limitation, and boundaries. That is actually what discipline means. Discipline is also discipleship: learning from a teacher. We are the teachers. Every adult teaches children about the world.

I first learned about giving form and limitation to children and creating boundaries for them when I was single and teaching emotionally handicapped children. It was during the sixties when the Summerhill approach to the education of children was popular. The essence of that approach is that we need to be free and children need to be free. If we control anything, then we are taking away a person's freedom. As a teacher, I used this approach for a while and had the children running all over the place doing whatever they wanted. I began to see that this total freedom was not good for them or for me. I was about to be fired and the children did not seem to be happy or free when they were running around. Actually they were running around in a great deal of misery.

So, I set up an individual program with each of them.

I gave each child a form for their learning experience during the day. The form consisted of a schedule within which they could do their reading, writing, and arithmetic. I told them they could arrange their subjects any way they wanted. They could put art in the form if they liked, they could do math all day, they could do whatever they wanted to do within the form since I was still being influenced by the freedom approach.

For the next three months they did everything that was on their lists. They would not change a thing even though they had that option. I experienced them as being so free and so happy that it blew all my theories about children and set me on a new path of understanding. I was experiencing freedom from these children within a strict form and all the time I had thought that formlessness was freedom.

Now I understand that form is the feminine quality, the quality of earth. If a building does not have form, it will collapse. A building gives us protection from the wind, rain, and cold. And yet, we get to freely experience everything that is outside of the building when we are inside of the building, like the sound of the raindrops and the sight of the snow.

As time went on, the children, who ranged from the ages of about nine to thirteen, started to add a little more art to their lists. All along I was expecting them to do art all day. What they were actually doing was more and more reading, writing, and spelling.

Finally, when the year was just about over, the forms were gone and the children were on their own schedules. They had their own self-control. It was totally unheard of for these emotionally handicapped children to behave so maturely and with so much enthusiasm for learning.

At the end of the year, the school gave these children tests and all the children went up three grade levels. At the beginning, these children did not even know how to write. Nobody was expecting that much achievement. It was a minor miracle for everyone who observed the process.

A similar thing happened at our Alive Polarity location in Calistoga in the children's group. I had a fence built around the play area to keep the children out of the street. The children, mostly between the ages of one and two years old, would run up to the fence, throw their toys over the fence, and then run back to where the main play area was. Then we would go over, pick up the toys, and put them back within the boundary.

After a while we decided to bring some of the toys back and leave some of them on the other side. The children began to get the idea that if they wanted to play with the toys, they were to stop throwing them over to the other side. Still, the children would throw their toys over the fence.

We got to thinking that the children wanted to go further than the fence since they kept throwing their toys over it. We also worried that they would run into the street where they might get killed if the fence was not there and we gave them their freedom.

This all went on for about a month or so until we decided to put in a lawn since the area we had enclosed was all pavement. In order to cut out a space in the pavement and put in the grass, we had to take down the fence. After we took the fence down, we let the children go outside. An amazing thing happened. The children stayed right where the fence used to be. Maybe ten or fifteen feet further back, nevertheless, still in the same area. They did not even want to wander out beyond the old boundaries. And what was even stranger to me was that they were still throwing their toys as if the fence was there!

I learned that when we "take the fence down," the fence will still be there, even though the physical form of the fence is gone. The children knew what their boundaries were, and through this knowledge they were learning about the positivity of limitation and what life is all about.

What I saw was that young children have a great desire for order and form. They really like to be told what their limitations are. Children learn how to have order and form within themselves from the limitation and form that is created for them on the outside. When children have that strong order and discipline on the outside, it eventually develops on the inside. Then they begin to discipline themselves. If we, as parents, start out by creating form and limitation for our children when they are very young, we will not be chasing our kids all over the place when they are thirteen.

So, if we think we can be "free" as human beings, we are fooling ourselves. We are imprisoned simply by being within the limits of our own bodies. People who do not accept the limitation of being in a body will commit suicide to gain their freedom. What I want to tell you is, people who commit suicide are not free. The thing we need to understand is that we have these weird space suits called bodies so we can be in this world; this is the basic limitation that we need to accept.

The other part we need to understand is that we can go overboard and get so obsessed with our form and body that we think we really are the body. Actually, the body is dead. What gives the body life is the soul emanating through the breath when we are born. The soul is the energy, it is the life spark, it is the sun, it is the light. When we get caught up thinking that our body is our soul, we are making a big mistake and we are losing a lot. The soul is not the body.

Once again, children know exactly the energy of what is going on and will usually admit to it when confronted with firm discipline and love. There was a young woman with two sons at an Alive Polarity Basic program. One day, during the question and answer period, the mother told me that her two and a half year old son objected to going to the children's group while she went to class. She knew that the boy had experienced a good deal of fighting between her and her husband, so she told him she went to class to learn how to be a better wife and mother.

The next day the child woke up and demanded that his mother not go to class. He cried, "I don't want you to stop fighting with Daddy. I want you to fight with Daddy." His mother told me she was shocked. She could hardly believe her ears, and yet she knew the boy was telling the truth. She was afraid to tell her son that she was angry with him for what he had said. She did not know how to deal honestly with her child.

Now here we have a classic example of how a child is literally begging for discipline and limitations. The boy is two and a half years old and he is acting like a fifty year old man, like a husband to his mother. That is what happens, that is exactly what happens! Children have the consciousness of an adult but they do not have the perspective of being an adult. After all, children are not having a sexual relationship, they are not birthing children, they do not know anything about that part of life. What parents can do is to give children guidelines on how to live as children in an adult world.

In this story we have a little boy running his mother's life, and ruining it as well, because she is letting him. We wonder how our children become so insecure. They become insecure because they have all this power that they really don't want. Furthermore, they have no idea how to use this power to deal with the world. Consequently, they feel very insecure.

What we need to accept is that children have already been patterned by our previous actions. After all, children copy us. We are their main teachers. When we finally focus and concentrate our energy towards our children so we can discipline them with clarity, all our old patterns will be regurgitated up in our faces because we created those patterns. We then have the opportunity to re-teach our children, share where we stand with them, and really be with them.

What we are doing is letting children know where we stand so they know their boundaries. The children will know somehow, deep inside, in spite of any reaction, that we love them. By talking honestly to our children, they will know exactly what we are thinking and feeling. There will be no confusion or guesswork on their part about what is going on. This clarity is a truly valuable gift we can give to our children. We can then teach our children to verbalize and share their feelings clearly, as well as give them the security of knowing the part they play in the whole family picture.

Now, children often react automatically from their emotional patterns. In order to find their limitations, they test us for our reaction. So what we can do is give discipline. Some children have more consciousness and less emotion, so they need less discipline. Others are very emotional and have very little conscious mind, so they need more limitation. When children accept limitation, they gain more consciousness and their boundaries broaden as their consciousness grows.

One of the questions that often comes up around the issue of discipline is how physical discipline, or spanking, fits into the form. Actually, physical discipline is the essence of form because form is physical. When we do something that is physical, it creates form. The best place to create form is the rear end. The gluteus is one of the negative poles of the brain. When the mind is caught in a particular negativity or resistance, resisting something that is positive, the rear end is the best place to apply physical energy.

A swift spank, with our full attention, with all of our focus, stimulates the negative pole. This brings all the energy and blood that is stuck up in the head down to the buttocks, the negative pole. The Aries energy is in the head. It is like a ram stubbornly ramming its horns, just the way children do when they do not get what they want. Children are stubborn, just like adults. They have as much power as we do. By spanking them, we are creating a form for them to learn how to be in the world.

So, a good spanking, maybe three swats that are very clear and penetrating, communicates to the child that we really mean what we are saying. Immediately the child's negative energy, that is stuck up in the Aries head, will move downwards in the body through all the other signs of the zodiac. This kind of discipline is not meant to hurt the child; only the child's pride, perhaps. Pride gets stuck up in the neck. Even though children may be small, when they get prideful they get all puffed up. Watch children when they are like that. Children will be just like adults when they get prideful.

By giving those swats, the pride gets broken and the energy moves down to the buttocks. Children realize the physical form we are creating for them. They feel our love. They really do want us to teach them how to be in this world.

Children get frustrated when they cannot do the same things we do. We can see this frustration especially in young children. One of the most frustrating times for them is when they are watching other children walk and they are not able to yet. They get angry, frustrated, and negative because they do not accept where they are. So by giving them a clear swat, they experience relief and grati-tude when they feel that form, that physical contact, and they are happy.

When spanking children, it is best to verbalize exactly what is going on. Even if children react and get resentful, it is important that we give their minds the understanding at the same time as the physical discipline and not later. We need to let children know what they are being spanked for, then and there, and give them all of our energy and focus at that moment.

An example of how I learned about focus and concentration was when I was teaching kindergarten as a single man. It was my first year and I was just learning how to be a teacher. In my class there was a five year old black boy who had the whole class wrapped around his little finger. He was the power in the class. Everyone else had to come to him to ask his permission when they wanted to do anything. This unwritten rule extended to teachers, as well.

One day when the class was in the playground, I saw that the boy was seeking reactions from other people. He was coming from his emotions and testing people. He was seeking reactions to find out how far he could go until someone would give him a limit.

So what happened was the boy came right up to me and kicked me in the knee really hard. At that point his demand was so great that I had to respond. I realized that I had been holding back when I was teaching because the boy had maintained control over the class. Now he was forcing me to give him attention and limitation.

I turned around and gave him, with energy and focus, a good "whack" on his bottom. Of course, the boy started to cry. He went over to a nearby wall and wailed for about twenty minutes.

The entire playground was stunned. We were all in a kind of shock. At the end of play period I blew my whistle and everyone, including the boy, went into the classroom. The boy went over and wailed in a corner. I started to teach the other children about words and colors when suddenly his crying stopped. He came over to me, climbed up on my lap, and listened to the rest of the lesson. It was a real revelation to me.

The next day his mother called me. She said, "What have you done to Jack?" I thought to myself, "Oh, my God." Then she said, "It's amazing. He's listening, sitting down, not wetting his bed, doing things for other people, and talking politely. I've never heard a polite word come out of his mouth before!"

I said, "Well, he kicked me in the knee and I spanked him." She replied, "You're the first person who's ever spanked him and earned his respect, too." So I realized that we had karma together. The spanking incident was meant to happen so we could both learn from it. Even though I was not his parent, I gave him my total energy. From that experience I learned how much children appreciate receiving an adult's conscious and focused attention. I learned how to give children exactly what they need and what they ask for before they react. It is like feeding milk to babies. We know when they are going to react, so we feed them at regular hours so they do not throw a tantrum. Anticipating their needs keeps the frustration level down for everyone.

The situation today is that many people have lost the understanding of how to love. They think that giving discipline to children is not giving love. Most of us feel love as attachment, when actually true love comes out of consciousness. If we are conscious, then there is real love, which is spiritual love. If we are reacting out of anger, confusion, and unclarity, then there is no love.

I can give you an example of how discipline is love.

This became very obvious with Marie, again. At first her parents were giving her lots of verbal direction, more of the air instead of the earth, the physical, which she could actually feel and understand. Then they started giving her more spankings, more physical discipline, especially because she is a Taurus and needs that earthiness. This physical discipline has made Marie feel more secure. In other words, her parents were actually giving her too much energy for her mental development when they were reasoning with her. By giving her the physical, the spanking, she was able to feel her boundaries and form at the moment of discipline and that gave her more security.

Many of us think, "Oh, I can't spank children. I'll traumatize their development. I'll hurt them." This rationale is usually coming from a place of weakness in the parents rather than from a place of strength. Parents need to be observers of what their children need at any time. From the attitude of an observer, parents can allow their children to reach a certain level of independence and can facilitate a new level of detachment.

When we discipline out of love, we are actually doing children a favor. Many people make the mistake of thinking that discipline, especially physical discipline, is punishing and hurtful rather than directive and guiding. It is no surprise that we have this misunderstanding because, actually, most of the time parents are spanking out of anger. It is definitely not the time to spank a child when we are angry. Then we pass on our anger and not our love. The purpose of discipline is not to vent our anger and frustration. It is to give our love. Otherwise, we will just keep perpetuating a vicious cycle of disease patterns.

For example, let's say a child, about one and a half, throws temper tantrums or cries whenever its mother leaves. This is the best time to work on the level of attachment between the mother and child so that the child can become more and more confident on its own. This is the time for firmness and clarity from both parents. If the mother is not clear in her own mind whether she actually wants to help in the process of detaching, whether she really wants to let go of the child needing her, then her confusion and hesitation will be transmitted to the child no matter what she says. It will be her energy, not her words, that comes through loud and clear. She will be giving double messages when what she says and what she feels are two different things. Then, anger and frustration will arise in both the mother and the child due to the lack of clarity. Any discipline which follows will be futile.

We need to realize how the mind traps us. The mind is a machine like a computer. The mind is totally neutral. All of our responses in life have been programmed. We do the same negative things over and over again out of habit. The mind, as well as the body, is part of our form here on earth, and form has to have a certain degree of negativity in it in order for it to exist in the first place.

So, because of all the worldly negativity, the mind is negatively patterned and grooved and becomes our enemy. What pulls us out of the groove is the soul. Our soul is positive. Our soul wants to do its work, give us life, and be alive and active in the body. The soul wants and needs that activity. The soul does not like to be ruled by the mind. The soul is chained by the body and the mind. It has become trapped in the mind's negative thoughts, forms, and patterns. Paradoxically, at any time, the soul can consciously change the computer that is inside us, in our mind and emotions. The soul can pierce through the computer because it is positive, totally enlightened, conscious and free. Any time we are conscious of what we are doing, even if we are doing something negative, it is the soul that is activating us.

God activates the soul and the soul starts pushing the mind, pushing us into a lot of negativity all at once, which creates a reaction. Then we are able to feel our pain. Sometimes the soul will have us do something that is very negative. It will push us down into the snake pit so we know there are snakes down there. It works in the same way as when adults let children get hurt; not letting them hurt themselves badly but allowing them to feel enough pain so they will become conscious of a dangerous situation and change their negative computer patterns.

By feeling the pain, we can stop doing the negative acts that we have been doing. We experience this process as painful when, in actuality, it is the positive action of God working through the soul changing the mind patterns of an individual. For instance, some people may be going deeper and deeper into a situation that is negative. Then, as they get to the place where it is really painful, they experience the pain completely, go through it, and totally change their lives.

This switch was the case with Mary Magdalene, the prostitute, when she became the beloved disciple of the Lord, Jesus Christ. Therefore, we cannot condemn anybody because we never know if they are really being negative, or if they are being pushed towards the positivity by going totally into their negativity.

Look at what is happening to so many young people today. They have slept around, taken drugs, and destroyed their bodies in many different ways. At the same time, their souls are starting to rise up like the phoenix out of the ashes. The freedom they are seeking is the quality of their higher selves, their souls. The soul says, "Okay, I'll give you what you think is freedom and let you experience it for awhile so that you can learn what real freedom is."

The mind is our enemy. It needs to be re-programmed. The mind will lure us with pleasures to keep us away from knowing our soul quality, our pain, and the experience of being detached and free. The mind continually wants to attach, attach, attach to more things and more pleasures. If it fails to attach to the pleasure, it wants to attach to more pain, but not enough pain so that we will surrender. The soul wants us to let go of the pain because the soul experiences no pain. Only the mind experiences pain. As we go through the pain, the soul, acting as a particle of the Lord, activates and pushes us towards the light, towards consciousness.

What is happening now, in this country, is that we are encouraging the development of our children's minds and totally forgetting about their emotional and physical development. Their mental, emotional, and physical bodies are not balanced with one another. In our schools, we emphasize increased mental growth in our children so we end up raising great computers. We teach algebra, calculus, and science earlier and earlier, which develops more mind and less intuition and feeling. We are molding our children to have great minds and they are emotional wrecks!

What happens to these children in the eighth grade, for example? We have all this birth control and still we have more and more pregnant girls. The reason is they want to get pregnant. These young girls want to feel that closeness, that womanhood. Psychologists and doctors say, "We don't get it. There are more teen-age pregnancies now, even with the pill, than ever before. It doesn't make sense."

Adults need to start recognizing that these young girls are feeling insecure. Teen-age girls do not have any idea how to deal with their sexual energy, their feelings, their emotions. These girls are not getting any help in school for this sort of thing because the emphasis is on increasing their mentality for college entrance. The schools teach respect for the mind, not for the feelings.

It is much the same story for boys in school. If it were not for sports in our country, the men would be total wimps. As it is, the brightest men in our country today are all up in their heads and have very little balance, if any, with their bodies or emotions. Their motor skill, the male energy, is given little, if any attention. Parents and schools have agreed upon encouraging the growth of the mind above all else. To get out of their heads and into their bodies and their feelings, boys need discipline, form, and strength.

Our children are learning that the way to escape their feelings and emotions is to become more mental. So they get more and more academic, go to more advanced classes, and skip grades while their emotional level stays the same. They escape their pain because they are focused up in their heads, their minds, while their pain is in their emotions and their physical bodies. Mental focus encourages children to become more and more separate within themselves and from each other.

My daughter, Liza, is very mental, as is my wife Sharon. Sharon and Liza have strong bodies, as well. Sharon's emotions are not as stable as her mind and neither are Liza's. So you can see, "Like mother, like daughter." As an experiment, I told Liza that I did not want to see an "A" on her report card. I told her to go out and have a good time. I was focusing less on her mentality and working on increasing her emotional and physical development.

Right now, in particular, Liza is getting closer and closer to me. I am giving her all my focus and clarity with firmness and love, through my discipline, which then gives her the form to help her live more easily in the world. I am teaching her how to deal with her feelings, something she does not learn in school. She is seeing what it is to be an adult, as well as what it is to have a healthy relationship with a strong and directive father, her male model.

Liza is in the eighth grade and we are working with her sexuality. We find dirty books she gets from her peers. We talk about them and ask her what she knows about sex. We communicate with her about men and her sexual feelings towards them, so when the time comes for her to focus with a man, her energy will be clear. I find it interesting that in my generation it was the boys who were running after the girls' skirts. Now, the girls' masculine energy is so out of balance, the girls are running after the guys' "skirts." There is a huge upsurge of homosexual energy in both sexes because of the imbalances that were created in the previous generations.

What I am doing with Liza is really being strong with her by giving her a lot of my male energy and a lot of my direction. In school, she was being teased by some rough girls who were very out of balance emotionally and very male. You see, Liza is tall, and she wanted to wear those tight pants and fairly high heels that are in fashion these days. I flatly refused. "You have a Pisces moon," I said, "you need to keep your feet on the ground."

I wanted her to look soft and feminine rather than hard and tough. Those tight pants automatically draw attention to the buttocks and genitals, which is sexual rather than feminine and graceful. The tightness of the pants and the height of the heels make it virtually impossible for girls to walk or to breathe correctly.

So, the rough girls would tease Liza for wearing low-heeled shoes and pretty skirts. They were actually teasing her for looking beautiful. All the teasing got to Liza and she started doing a big "poor-me" about not being allowed to wear tight pants and high-heels. She was feeling, "Oh, poor-me, I have to wear all these pretty clothes."

One day I asked Liza, "Is it the boys that tease you about wearing pretty skirts or just the girls?"

She paused and smiled, "Only the girls," she said. "In fact, the boys like the way I dress. They're definitely attracted to me." Then she realized what I had seen all along. The girls were teasing Liza out of jealousy and, maybe, for some of them, unconscious homosexual feelings. It was not that they thought she looked funny at all. Actually, it was just the opposite. Liza was so attractive, she had upset their dominance and power. The girls were using their sexual energy in a negative way to control who got the attention.

These girls kept up the teasing and Liza became more and more emotional. So, finally I said, "Okay, I want you to come to me every morning and I'll check your shoes, your skirt, and everything you are wearing. From now on, I'm going to tell you exactly what to wear and what I want you to do."

In the morning she got dressed, put on her nicest skirt and shoes, and came in looking really pretty. I said, "Oh, Liza, you look beautiful." I gave her a hug and she went off to school feeling really good. I created a very strong form for her because she was an emotional wreck from the stress of the teasing and the feelings that were coming up for her.

I also knew that Liza wanted to be "Miss Popular" in her class so I said to her, "Look, you are in a very unique situation. Here in Calistoga (the Alive Fellowship owns and operates the Alive Polarity Inn, a vegetarian health resort) you have a "family-pub." You can bring all your friends over here and you can socialize with non-alcoholic malt beverages and fancy grape juices. You can even have a dance if you want to. You aren't thinking of any of that."

"So," I said, "I'm ordering you to give me a list of the five most popular children in your class and we'll invite them here for dinner with all the special treats of the house. They can do anything they want. They can even go into the Jacuzzi and go swimming, too. I've switched and put myself into your situation and these are the things I would do if I were you. These are the things I am ordering you to do."

When Liza came home the next day I asked her if she was still being teased and she said, "Oh, no, not at all." When I asked her what was happening she said, "I told some of the kids about the party and they were all really excited about it. So, now I'm completing my list of the most popular kids in the class." Then she came up to me and squeezed me. Due to my direction, she was able to feel really close to me.

What I am doing for Liza is teaching her what a man is. As she gets closer to me she is really feeling my energy. When men begin to be attracted to her, she will have the ability to choose between the positive or negative ones and find another strong and gentle man like her father.

By giving Liza a strong form with narrow boundaries, I am helping her to be happy. After the form has been built, I can tear it down. There is no need for boundaries anymore. Happiness can be taught to our children. Learning how to be positive with what is given is one of the greatest gifts we can pass on to our children. Acceptance, a very basic lesson in life, is learned from the parents. Once again, we reflect our parents and our children reflect us.

Another very important lesson, and one which usually is very hard for us to learn, is how to discriminate what course of action needs to be taken in different life situations. We usually teach our children, as we were taught, to stand up for their principles no matter what. Instead of teaching our children to assess the individual situation and respond consciously to what is called for, we are teaching them to go for a reaction. This problem of lack of discrimination comes up over and over and over again for teenagers, as well as for adults.

Here's a beautiful example of what I mean. Liza has been learning how to play tennis in her P.E. class at school. She knows all the rules, her body is becoming more coordinated, and she is becoming a good tennis player. One day, a school tournament was set up and Liza was playing opposite the same rough girls who teased her about her clothes. Their idea of how to play tennis was if they hit the ball over the net onto Liza's side, they got a point. All they were really saying to Liza was, "You don't get any points and we get all the points."

So, Liza, knowing the game, said, "Oh, no, that isn't how to play the game," and proceeded to tell them how they were wrong. She was being very mental with very rough girls in an emotional situation. They countered by insisting on their way. Liza was getting frustrated because she was not winning, so she went to the teacher and told her that these girls did not know how to play the game. The teacher came over to watch and sure enough the girls were still playing their own way. The teacher said, "You're not playing the game correctly. Go take four laps around the field." Then she told Liza, "Don't worry, Liza, if they do this again with you or if you have any trouble with them, I'll kick them out of my class."

Well, that was wonderful for the teacher. Then the teacher wouldn't have to deal with the girls anymore. It was terrible for Liza, because Liza was with them in other classes and lived with them in the same town. So, the girls got furious with Liza, they harassed her, and pushed her into the lockers. They were angry because they did not win their game and they had to run four laps, all because of Liza.

When Liza came home and told me this story, I was ready to go to the principal and talk to the girls' parents and all that until I questioned Liza more fully and more details emerged.

Then I said to her, "Your mentality was not dealing with the emotions. You did not want to let them win because you wanted to win so badly. You wanted to play the game the "right way." You were being Miss Uppity and telling them what to do. So you blew it. You were being an intellectual bully, which is no better than the other girls."

Liza said, "I don't understand."

I said, "Do you want to be beaten up? Go get beaten up, then. You're calling it on yourself."

"I don't understand."

"Okay, what would have happened if you just played the game and let them win?"

"Well, they would have won!"

"Would they have beaten you up?"

"No."

"What would have happened after that?"

"Well, they would have gone up in the tournament and they would have played another match."

"Do you think they would have played the same way?"

"Yes."

"Do you think that somewhere along the line the teacher would find out the way they were playing and it would be very clear to her that they didn't know how to play tennis?"

"Oh, yeah."

"So, what do you need to do?"

"I need to apologize to those girls."

"That's exactly right. Apologize for being Miss Uppity."

So Liza went to the girls and said, "You were right about how to play a tennis game. You hit the ball over the net and you get a point. I was totally wrong. Your way was right and I apologize for being Miss Smarty."

This totally blew the girls' minds. None of the other children had ever done that with them before. One of the girls even told Liza that she appreciated her for coming over and apologizing. Liza was not beat up anymore and in a week both girls were kicked out of school anyway.

See, everybody involved knew the truth of the matter. The girls knew they were lying and Liza knew they were violent. So, if Liza had used that information and agreed with them, instead of setting up an opposition, a polarity, then she would not have attracted their reaction. This kind of situation is very subtle, yet it is a common one we all have to deal with at various times during our lives. We need to see how we attract negative energy to ourselves by not being discriminating with the response that is appropriate in an individual situation.

Instead of placing ourselves in opposition to someone and creating a polarity because we think we know the "right way," we can agree with them instead. We can realize that someone may be negative and may hurt us no matter what we do. We usually say, "Oh, no, that's wrong, I know the right way." Those are the times when our intellect and our uppityness do not allow us to deal with the real situation at hand. In this case, it was Liza being confronted by two violent people. Usually our ego tells us other people are wrong, and then we become violent ourselves. Instead of helping the situation, our opposition makes us the same as our opponents. When we set up an opposition to violence, we will immediately find ourselves in a violent situation.

By agreeing, we learn humility. We can use the truth of any situation to avoid violence. The girls were looking for disagreement. They also wanted to win. So instead of disagreeing, we can let them win. When there is agreement, there is no polarity, no reaction set up. Whoever is being provocative will look elsewhere for the disagreement because there is no longer any energy in the situation. We are usually so hooked into being "right," we lose sight of when to duck.

This is a vital lesson for us all, not just teenagers. As we grow more conscious, gradually we will stop going for a reaction in another person. When another person is looking for disagreement, looking for a fight, we can switch the energy by having compassion for the other person's pain. We can give them the opportunity to break their negative mind pattern by agreeing with them. That way, we take the wind out of their sails and dissipate the negative energy.

For people who are married, the same principle follows. We know if we say a certain thing, we can get a reaction from our partner. So, we can either keep our mouth shut, or say it. Most of us say it because we like the reaction. As we get more conscious, the emotion lessens, and we let go of needing to go for the reaction.

Learning when to agree and when to disagree is an important part of discrimination. When I was a reservist in the Marine Corps, the drill instructor thought I was heavy and came up to me and said, "I'm sending you to the fat farm." I did not want to go to the fat farm because it was a place where they run men into the ground, a small hell. So I disagreed with him. I said, "Sir, I'm not going to the fat farm. I can do twenty pull-ups." So I did thirty and he never bothered me again.

In other words, I knew that I could give him what he was looking for. He needed strong men in his platoon so that he could win the medals he wanted. By knowing the truth of the situation, I was able to use it to give him what he wanted. He was trying to get rid of me because he thought I was a fat weakling. I showed him that I was able to be even more than what he wanted.

So, another part of discrimination is knowing the appropriate response in any given situation and being conscious enough not to need to be right. Then we allow a clear response rather than an emotional reaction or an intellectual rationale. It is all part of accepting what is happening. If the wind is going against us, all the insisting in the world is not going to change its course. Consciousness is learning to discriminate between the times when we can change what is being given to us, and the times when we need to accept what is being given. Mutability is the primary rhythm of life.

This rhythm of mutability is what parenting is all about. A parent-teacher is in a constant state of re-examining his or her own consciousness and understanding. Life is change. As we gain more awareness through our own experience, we learn the basic lessons of living in this world. When we remain open to our own life lessons, we can pass on our consciousness and positivity to our children at any given moment. Then we know we are doing the best we can do. Our impetus to become clear is not only for our own growth and development as souls, but for the evolving consciousness of our children.

Let's remember that we are all parents and we are all children. We are all parents to one another. We are on this earth to help one another reflect the truth. Our work is to mirror each other with clarity, consciousness, and love. Only then will we begin to understand the meaning of true spirituality.

GLOSSARY

— A —

action
All our thoughts and actions will be met with equal and opposite reactions in our future. Action is the creative, masculine half of the Law of Karma.

air element
The main element of the fourth chakra, centered in the chest. The emotional quality of the air element is desire, and its main physical quality is speed.

air principle
The neutral aspect of energy, existing at the balance point between positive and negative; neither male nor female; it carries prana, the life force, into the physical world. The air principle is a reflection of the One energy of pure spirit before it splits into the three principles of air, fire, and water in its descent into the physical world.

Akashic Record

The account of all our actions and reactions, existing on the astral plane.

ALIVE

An acronym, A Living Inner Vitality Experience.

Alive Fellowship

An organization established by Jefferson Campbell to provide a strong foundation for the Alive Polarity health programs. Members of the Fellowship live according to the teachings of Alive Polarity.

astrology

The relationship between the body and celestial gravity.

astrological chart

A planetary graph of the potential for growth in consciousness of a particular soul in its lifetime.

astral plane or realm

One of the levels of existence, part of the mental realm. The astral plane is the first level above the physical body where the fire principle forms the emotions.

attachment

Emotional associations which cause us to move upwards or downwards into more positivity or negativity; the magnetic force of past associations which brings souls into the physical world. Attachment is the emotional quality of the water chakra, the chakra that also includes sexuality.

Awareness Counseling
A technique for self-understanding developed by Jefferson Campbell. It is unique in its emphasis on acceptance and forgiveness. Awareness Counseling is a powerful tool for learning how to be positive.

— B —

birth
The moment in life when the first breath is taken and prana activates the five elements that are latent in the womb; our first realization of the outer world.

bi-polar current
A flow of energy in the body, moving in a spiralling motion from head to toe and left to right, created by the water principle.

body
A "space suit" taken on by the soul so it can exist at the physical level and communicate with other souls. We are not the body: the body is an image, a reflection of who we really are. It is a slowed-down vibration of energy, an illusion.

boundaries
Clearly defined limits for behavior, providing security and consistency in relationships. For children, boundaries provide an opportunity for learning and discipline.

— C —

causal plane or realm

The second level above the physical, where our past actions provide the blueprint for our present mental patterns.

Chakra

One of the seven energy centers in the body in which energy is transformed as it moves downwards into slower and denser vibrations. The seventh chakra, at the crown of the head, is spiritual. The sixth, at the eye center or pineal gland, is mental. The bottom five are physical and are located at the throat (ether), chest (air), solar plexus (fire), pelvis (water), and rectum (earth). The chakras are the centers from which each emotion radiates to create the physical body.

consciousness

Awareness of soul quality, the degree to which the soul is liberated from the domination of the mind and emotions.

conception

The moment when the soul enters the physical plane and the polarity of the mother and father. Conception is the moment when we come under the influence of our first two teachers, our parents.

crystallization

The tendency of energy to slow down and create form as it descends from pure spirit to the physical plane.

— D —

death
The moment of transition when the soul departs the physical plane. The soul never dies.

destiny
Our situation in life, resulting from our past actions. The most spiritual word in Western language for the law of action and reaction, called karma in the East.

detachment
Breaking negative bonds of association by consciously attaching to the positive spiritual qualities in ourselves and others.

devotion
Giving; selfless service and love; appreciating that everything is a gift from the Lord. Devotion is a main quality of the receptive feminine energy.

disease
The crystallization of negative emotions in the body resulting from focusing on the negative aspects of our life situations.

duality
Polarity, Yin-Yang; the existence of opposites: heaven-earth, positive-negative, day-night, pleasure-pain, man-woman, love-hate, good-bad, action-reaction.

— E —

earth
The planet represents the feminine energy, receptive to heaven and nourishing all life.

earth element
The main element of the first and densest chakra, centered at the rectum. The emotional quality of earth is fear, and its main physical quality is bones.

elements
At the physical level, the five aspects of energy which compose physical matter. In descending order, from the lightest to the densest, the elements are ether, air, fire, water and earth.

elimination
A surfacing and expelling of negativity, caused by moving our energy and increasing our vibration through positivity.

emotional alchemy
Using consciousness to change mental habits and disease patterns, transforming negative emotional patterns to positive ones.

emotions
Our unconscious, intangible qualities of grief, desire, anger, attachment, and fear. The emotions create the physical body. Emotions can pull us upwards or downwards, depending on whether they are positive or negative.

energy
The powerful cosmic vibration that permeates all creation. It starts as a purely spiritual force and moves down through levels of increasing density to create, sustain, and destroy all lower levels of the universe. It has many names, but in essence it is indescribable.

ether
The element of space, the center of the emotions on the physical plane, located at the throat chakra. Its main physical quality is grief: the longing for escape from duality, and for reunion with God. The ether is the highest physical chakra in the body, and grief is the highest emotion.

— F —

feminine qualities
In both men and women, the ability to be receptive, devotional, nurturing, mutable, yielding and reflective.

fire element
The main element of the third chakra, centered at the solar plexus. The emotional quality of fire is anger and its main physical quality is hunger.

fire principle
The creative, positive aspect of energy, called Raja, in the Vedas. It is the masculine energy that dominates the astral level of action.

fool

Being vulnerable, taking risks: it is necessary to be able to be the fool and risk the ridicule of those to whom we are attached in order to break out of negative patterns.

form

In nature, the structure of energy crystallized on the physical plane; in human relationships, boundaries we set for living.

freedom

Real freedom is understanding that the soul is imprisoned in this world of limitation.

free will

Our attitude; this attitude determines our actions which create future reactions that will reflect our positivity or negativity.

— H —

healing

Increased positivity resulting from our male and female energies coming into balance. Healing is consciousness; it happens when we take responsibility for ourselves and our actions.

healing crisis

The surfacing of negativity that occurs when consciousness is increased at the physical, emotional, or mental levels. The soul's energy speeds up and drives out the lower vibrations of negativity which appear to us as symptoms of disease. "Crisis" refers to the occurrence of these symptoms which tests our determination to be positive.

heaven
The symbol of the male energy in nature. The sun and sky pour out heat and light into creation. This energy is the action that makes all reactions possible.

higher mind
Conscious mind. The higher mind operates when we manifest our soul qualities of courage, forgiveness, devotion, and surrender, and use our power to attach to God, the truth, in each person.

homeopathic principle
The phenomenon of "like attracts like"; we attract people and events with a vibration similar to our own.

humility
Accepting our diseases, accepting how and where we've made mistakes. Humility comes when God, the soul, forces the mind to see its limitations.

husband
A woman's marriage partner; a reflection of her own male energy, giving her an opportunity to accept her masculine side, her secondary energy.

— I —

idea
A mental blueprint for future form.

I-Ching or Book of Changes
An ancient Chinese philosophical text giving an understanding of life. The *I-Ching* is probably the most accessible ancient text for Westerners to read and understand.

intellectual knowledge
Knowing by objective logic and reason; the masculine, scientific, and complex side of the mind.

intuitive knowledge
Knowing by subjective experience, perceiving subtle qualities; the animal part of the mind that can feel nature; the feminine, simple side of the mind.

— K —

Karma
The inescapable law of action and reaction; the chain of past actions, associations, and attachments which determines our present and future. "As you sow, so shall you reap."

— L —

life
The presence of God's vibration (breath, prana, energy) in a physical form.

life history
An account of our life which shows us our patterns of behavior. These patterns are important clues to how our male and female energies are out of balance and where, in the body, our energy is blocked.

limitation
The fact that we live in a human body in a world of opposites. We are not free, we are separate from God. We must accept our limitations to be in harmony with nature.

love
True human love is being attached only to the positive parts, the soul qualities, in another person. Spiritual love is totally selfless devotion to God.

lower mind
Unconscious mind. The lower mind is operating when we manifest our animal qualities of lust, anger, greed, attachment, and pride.

— M —

manipulation
Physically affecting the energy flow in the body by touch.

marriage
A lifelong commitment to the union of a man and a woman, giving both partners a constant reflection of their secondary energy and an opportunity to know and accept the "other half" of themselves.

masculine qualities
In men or women, the ability to be responsible, creative, outgoing, directive, truthful, and constructive.

meditation
Stilling the mind; looking inwards instead of outwards; the soul working towards reunion with God through inner contemplation.

mental realm or plane
The subtle level of existence between the physical world and the spiritual realm. It is here in the causal and astral regions that the soul is covered by the mind and emotions in its descent into the world.

mind
Our computer for functioning in the world, a blueprint for our lives, composed of our past actions.

mutability
The primary rhythm of life; flexibility, yielding, change-ability, avoiding polarization. Mutability is an important quality of the feminine energy.

— N —

nature
The laws and form of the physical world; also, a symbol of the feminine energy.

negativity
Emotions, unconsciousness, sense pleasures, disease; moving downwards, away from God and our soul quality.

nurturing
Nourishing, caring, encouraging growth; looking for and finding the life and positivity in others.

—O—

observer
Having a detached perspective, reflecting the neutral air principle; being able to distinguish our soul qualities from our body and mind.

—P—

pain
A blockage of energy and the main method of instruction in the school of life. Pain awakens us to our negativity.

patterns
Recurring situations or ways of behaving. Disease patterns are chronic inherited imbalances in our male and female energies which are repeatedly expressed in many areas of our lives. Awareness of our patterns can help us become more conscious of our imbalances.

physical plane or realm
The dense materialization of the mind, the lowest level of creation. On the physical plane, the soul is trapped by mind and matter.

physical body
The soul's vehicle for reincarnation. The characteristics of the body are a map of our destiny and of the lessons we need to learn in our lifetime.

pleasure
Sense stimulation which attaches us to the physical world. A free flow of energy in the body.

polarity
Duality, Yin-Yang; the existence of opposites: heaven-earth, positive-negative, day-night, man-woman, love-hate, good-bad, action-reaction. Polarity is the fundamental way the mind is able to make sense of the world. We know something only in distinguishing it from its opposite or absence.

"poor-me"
Irresponsibility: not accepting our situations in life, not realizing they are all our own creation and the results of our past actions.

positivity
Moving upwards to a higher vibration, becoming more conscious and less emotional, expressing soul qualities.

Prana
The "breath of life"; energy moving through the air principle to give life to physical form.

principles
The three aspects of the One energy as it manifests in the mental and physical realms; the triune function, or Trinity. The three principles are air (neutral), fire (positive), and water (negative).

psychic energy
The power we have to function on the astral plane. Using psychic energy is very damaging and depleting to our vitality and causes us to lose our spiritual attainments.

— R —

Raja
(From Sanskrit) The positive, masculine aspect of energy; the fire principle, creativity, action, motion, time.

reaction
The inescapable result of action; the feminine, reflective half of the Law of Karma.

receptivity
The ability to be devotional and nurturing; reflecting and complementing the masculine energy; accepting what comes to us. The quality of receptivity shows the health of the feminine energy in men or women.

reflection
Seeing ourselves in all situations and associations in our lives. We are all mirrors for each other.

reincarnation
The soul's repeated journeys to the physical plane. Our karmic attachments keep bringing us back to the world.

resistance
Non-acceptance; the difficulty encountered by energy moving in matter; the difficulty our soul has in expressing its qualities while under the domination of the mind.

responsibility
Being true to our word, the ability to respond truthfully to the reactions we create. Responsibility shows the health of the masculine energy in men or women.

— S —

Sattva

(From Sanskrit) The air principle, the neutral balance point between male (Raja) and female (Tamas). The Sattva is a reflection of the spiritual realm: harmony, well-being, neutral observation, understanding, peace.

Saturn cycle

The planet Saturn in our astrological chart shows how we will be tested and where we will meet constriction in our lives. Every fourteen years, from the time of our birth, Saturn is either in opposition to, or has returned to, its natal position in the chart. These are commonly known as the "Saturn Opposition" and "Saturn Return." These times are significant points of transition, when our negativity or positivity will be amplified and made more obvious by painful or joyful events.

seeking

Looking for a teacher; spiritually, the soul's longing for freedom from the domination of the mind, longing for reunion with God.

soul

The imperishable, spiritual aspect of ourselves that brings life to the body and mind. The soul is a particle of God which can enter the physical plane of action and reaction only by taking on a mind and body.

space

Another word for the ether element, which is centered in the fifth chakra at the throat. Its main emotional quality is grief. Space also refers to a quality of the feminine energy, the "empty stage" which provides a form for action, the masculine energy.

spiral
The shape of energy as it spins in the world.

spirit
Soul quality, energy; a particle of God.

surrender
Total humility and acceptance of grief, a point in our growth when we realize we are nothing and fall on our knees asking the Lord for help. Surrender is the opposite of pride.

switch
A moment of transition when we break out of a habitual pattern, moving from one attitude to its polar opposite.

— T —

Tamas
(From Sanskrit) The negative, feminine aspect of energy in the physical world; the water principle, reaction, elimination, coolness, space.

time
A never-ending unfolding of events caused by the fire principle through its qualities of action and motion. Timing is an important masculine quality.

transition

A critical moment which gives an opportunity for learning; a time when we use our positive energy for growth, acceptance, and understanding in a situation that could be very painful.

triune function

The Trinity, the three aspects of the One energy when it separates from pure spirit; the three principles of fire, air, water. Many names have been given to these aspects of energy: positive-neutral-negative; masculine-neuter-feminine; Action-Nothing-Reaction; Creator-Sustainer-Destroyer; Father-Son-Holy Ghost.

toxins

Crystallized negativity in the body. The body will absorb and hold negativity, gradually poisoning itself, if toxins are not eliminated.

transverse current

The spiral-shaped flow of energy down the spine, covering the body; the movement of the air principle in the body.

— U —

umbilical current

The spiral-shaped flow of energy radiating out from the umbilicus; the movement of the fire principle in the body.

— V —

Vedas
Ancient sacred books of India which give an understanding of life.

vibration
The subtle movement of energy in the body which speeds up when we are conscious and slows down when we are emotional. Our vibration is high when our present actions are positive. Thus we create future positive reactions.

vitality
Our stored reserve of inherited energy, the magnetism that unites the sperm and the egg in conception. There are two aspects of vitality: mental, as seen in the length of the earlobes, and physical, as seen in the firmness of the buttocks. Mental vitality helps us recognize our mistakes and learn from them; physical vitality helps us survive disease in the body and rebound to heal quickly.

— W —

water
Symbolizes the feminine energy: reflective, mutable, ever-changing, cyclical, nurturing, original source of all life on the physical plane.

water element
The main element centered in the pelvis, the second chakra. Its emotional quality is love or attachment. Its main physical quality is the fluid of reproduction, the semen in man and the egg in woman.

water principle
The receptive, negative aspect of energy, called Tamas in the Vedas; the feminine energy that dominates the physical level of reaction.

wife
A man's marriage partner who is a reflection of his own feminine energy, giving him an opportunity to accept his feminine side.

work
Doing our "work" means understanding and accepting our lessons in life.

Wu-Wei
In Taoism, the "effortless effort"; harmony with nature, balance between the receptive and the outgoing; a moment in the Sattva.

— Y —

Yin-Yang
The Oriental symbol of nature; a spiralling interaction of polar opposites, each containing the seed of, and becoming, the other. Yin-Yang illustrates the complementary natures of the male and female energies. Yin is feminine and Yang is masculine.

A Note about the Author

Jefferson Campbell was born in Pawtuckett, Rhode Island, in 1947. He has spent the last eight years teaching people how to use *Alive Polarity* to improve the quality of their lives. Graced with gifted hands, philosophical vision, and administrative abilities, Jefferson is a co-founder of the *Alive Polarity Programs* and serves as its President.

Jefferson earned his teaching credentials at Sonoma State College, where he majored in humanistic psychology. He is the creator of Awareness Counseling techniques and he pioneered the application of this method with emotionally handicapped children and delinquent adolescents. In addition, he counseled in the field of community mental health.

Looking for psycho-physical integration, Jefferson experienced Rolfing and Lomi body work before he studied with Dr. Randolph Stone, the founder of Polarity Therapy. Jefferson has absorbed and translated the essence of Dr. Stone's teachings into the process we know as *Alive Polarity.* Now his lectures have been transformed into this educational and personally useful book.

Alive Polarity
Program Information

This book has been created from lectures given during many of the classes that form our program entitled ''Healing Yourself and Your Family.'' This six-week program gives the practical knowledge that is the basis of all our Health and Self-Growth programs.

''Healing Yourself and Your Family'' is a program that will help you overcome the stress, pollution, and other tensions of modern living. At Alive Polarity's Murrieta Hot Springs, a vegetarian spa renowned for its curative mineral-rich waters, you'll find a natural oasis of rest, calm, and serenity. There are no phones, no televisions, and no deadlines; just glorious weather, spectacular scenery, and fresh clean air.

Current medical research reveals that increasing numbers of people, particularly those with stressful or sedentary lives, are showing a dramatic upswing of what health professionals call ''diseases of choice.'' These maladies include high blood pressure, overeating, chronic fatigue, lower back pain, lack of physical exercise, nervous disorders, and coronary artery disease.

The good news, however, is that most of these situations are preventable since everyone can do something about the state of their own health. Today, both men and women want to gain confidence in themselves mentally, emotionally, and physically. They are seeking a better understanding of their relationships and their individual health values are higher than ever before. Many make a strong connection between looking good and feeling good and want the benefits of the greater vitality that comes from exercising, good eating habits, and relief from stress.

It was with these ideals in mind that the program "Healing Yourself and Your Family" was created. Over the past seven years, this program has provided guests with the environment they need to get reoriented and reorganized, to sort out plans, and to become clearer for a more positive future. For many it is a time for renewal of the spirit. It is a chance for more self-knowledge and self-mastery. For couples, it's also a new way to explore the workings of marriage.

The varied interests and activities of the guests that form each group seem to spark the development of close new friendships. As feelings are shared with each other, companionship and support grow. The good-fellowship, both from the guests and the staff, gives everyone a special lift that helps fulfill personal goals.

Alive Polarity consists of four major elements: Emotional Awareness Counseling, Energy Balancing Body Sessions, PolarEnergetics postures, and dieting-fasting-cleansing. These techniques form a foundation which make it possible for our other classes and services to make their greatest impact.

The Awareness Counseling classes (there are 2 or 3 each week) are a penetrating way to get in touch with the positivity in any situation. They will help you to look at, and eliminate, the habits that are creating unwanted stress and tension in your life.

Doing an awareness can improve communications between you and other people.

Each week you'll receive an Alive Polarity Energy Balancing Body Session. You may choose from three kinds of touch that can be used either individually or in combination. Each of these touches will help recharge your vitality, balance your mental, emotional, and physical bodies, and lead to greater health and mental alertness.

Two additional features are Body Readings and Life Histories. In the Body Reading class, you'll learn how emotions actually create the physical body. You'll find out what your body is saying about you. In the Life Histories class, you will see how you repeat old patterns that may have led to the physical blocks mapped in your body reading. Both of these tools are used by your Staff Counselor to make your Awarenesses and Body Sessions more effective.

Hippocrates declared that regular exercise is man's best friend. Our daily PolarEnergetics classes comprise a complete regimen of postures that, like yoga, combine movement, stretch, sound, and breath in ways that will quickly help you feel better. There are theory classes that teach you how to use these postures at home. And, in addition, each week there are "Tone and Stretch" and "AquaEnergetics" exercise classes.

In the Alive Polarity food classes, we'll cover topics such as: the use of vitamins and herbs to supplement and build the body; vitality drink—an easy, functional way to cleanse the liver; wheatgrass juice and its detoxifying and healing qualities; the nutritional value of sprouts and easy ways to grow them; fasting and cleansing techniques to gain or lose weight and detoxify the body. You'll also learn about the vibrations of foods and gain a true understanding about the difference between being a meat eater and a vegetarian.

Whether you're single, married, or a parent, this program has something for everyone. We'll discuss how to handle your sexual energy and look at subjects such as celibacy, courting, engagement, and marriage. You'll learn how to express your positive male and female energies and thus attract the same positivity in other people. Other classes, touched upon in this book, include: Receptivity, Balancing the Male and Female Energies, Marriage and Family Dynamics, and Parenting.

This Alive Polarity program offers the opportunity to be away from familiar surroundings in a supportive environment. The facilities at Murrieta make this even more inviting. There is a men's and a women's spa that are each equipped with dressing facilities, Saunas, individual mineral baths (many with whirlpool equipment), and private rooms where you can enjoy Skin Glow Rubs, Herbal Wraps, Alive Polarity Body Sessions, massage, or relaxation in between baths. There are also two marvelous mud bath facilities, one for men and one for women, where you can take advantage of the famous Tule mud extracted from the mineral hot springs located on the property.

Outdoors you'll find three mineral pools. One is a large Roman Bath for lounging, another is a smaller pool for playing water volleyball and doing AquaEnergetics exercises, and the third is a beautiful, large pool with a fountain designed by the same gentlemen who gave us the outdoor pool at Hearst Castle.

There are also fourteen championship tennis courts (some with lights) surrounding a pro-shop and over 40 acres of grounds for longs walks and peaceful vegetarian picnics. Nearby there are public golf courses, as well as boating on Lake Elsinore. Along with the above services, we also offer Rebounder exercising, Backswing technique, European facial massage, Cellulite massage, internal cleansing, and Lymph massage.

Using energy to regenerate or heal is an ancient art. Alive

Polarity brings that art into the present where you can take advantage of the truth and wisdom that pervades these teachings. As your energy flow is re-established, your awareness of virtues like humility, selfless service, patience, integrity, and devotion are heightened. You'll return home rested and rejuvenated.

The classes associated with Alive Polarity principles and health practices are available at Alive Polarity's Murrieta Hot Springs. Additional services available include: room and board, Tule mud baths, private mineral baths, 3 outdor mineral pools, saunas, facials, massage, herbal wraps, Lymph massage, Skin Glow Rubs, Cellulite massage, tennis, and other miscellaneous health and spa activities. To receive a list of all the activities we offer and the latest rates, please contact our Murrieta Program Information Center.

We also offer Alive Polarity Seminars entitled, "Introduction to Healing Yourself and Your Family." At these seminars you will learn how to use Alive Polarity tools to improve your health, heal your emotions, and strengthen your family.

These seminars work with the emotional and physical stresses that can lead to health problems and affect your relationships. They are sponsored by previous guests of the six-week program and include experience in Awareness Counseling, Body and Pulse Reading, becoming a vegetarian, PolarEnergetics postures, and Energy Balancing Body Work.

Alive Polarity Seminars are being held all over the United States as well as in other parts of the world. If you would like to attend one of these seminars, please contact us and we will be pleased to send you information about the next seminar to be held in your area.

Over the years many of you have been kind enough to make donations to help us expand our teachings, services, and facilities. It is your financial support that has made it possible for us to help many people through the teachings of Alive Polarity principles and health practices. For those of you who have supported us by purchasing this book, we say a hearty thank you. We hope you will be stimulated to attend an Alive Polarity Health and Self-Growth program sometime soon. In the meantime any amount of money that you are able to donate will be helping people from throughout the world to heal themselves and their families. Please make your check payable to The Alive Fellowship. Again, thank you for your continuing support.

Patrons

Our special thanks to the following people for their timely support in the publication of this book

Mr. & Mrs. M.J. Abelsohn	Capetown, South Africa
Mr. & Mrs. Alex Allison	Encino, California
Michael & Lorena LaForest Bass	Ashland, Oregon
Willi B. Bauer	Brunn, Austria
Anne M. Bellak	Alexandria, Virginia
Stacia Bevan	Seattle, Washington
Linda Bresnan	Portland, Oregon
Claire Callan	London, England
Salvatore Caronna	Santa Rosa, California
Dr. & Mrs. Arthur Ben Chitty, Jr.	Sewanee, Tennessee
Jacqueline Clayton	Seattle, Washington
William Combi	Novato, California
John R. Cowell	Salt Lake City, Utah
Dean & Darcy	Seattle, Washington
Theo Donna	Santurce, Puerto Rico
Robert A. & Robyn L. Ellis	Poulsbo, Washington
Lynn Ellsworth	Fresno, California
Karen L. Emerick	S. Glastonbury, Connecticut
Barry and Cynthia Epstein	Lexington, Kentucky
Scot & Sharon Espy	Seattle, Washington
Face and Body Care (Betty J. Rostoni, Prop.)	San Rafael, California
Gary Flatt	Seattle, Washington
Charles & Claire Fox	N. Bellmore, New York
Albert Furniss	Oakland, California
Dennis & Barbara Garcia	Bellevue, Washington
Amelia Giusto	Middletown, California
Louise Gosho	Calistoga, California
Dan Grinde	Bigfork, Montana

Kenneth & Barbara Gulick	St. Helena, California
Steven & Ming Hall	San Lorenzo, California
Kay Herron	Los Angeles, California
Blanche F. Howard	North Palm Beach, Florida
Gail & Alan Hutcheson	Manchester, Missouri
Ardyce Hutmacher	San Francisco, California
Jay & Jamie Jedinak	Bellevue, Washington
Don & Susan Jensen	Fresno, California
Nicholas Jones	London, England
Pamela Christine Rhodes Jones	Ontario, Canada
Gordon & Marlyn Keating	Seattle, Washington
Liese A. Keon	Belvedere, California
Rod & Virginia Kirkwood	Seattle, Washington
Gary Land D.C.	Redding, California
Kathleen M. Lee	Wausau, Wisconsin
Phillip & Dorothy Lontz	Waitsfield, Utah
Mallat Family	Morongo Valley, California
Maggie Mansfield	London, England
Richard T. Marks	Nevada City, California
Don & Loris Maroney	Hacienda Heights, California
Gregory & Annie Martin	Lake Elsinore, California
Lucy Mayer	Baden, Austria
William D. Moody	Fairbanks, Alaska
Sylvia T. Moore	Gualala, California
Ron Morey	Atherton, California
Doug & Sheryl Newland	Eugene, Oregon
Norman H. Nisly	Alta Loma, California
Dan & Elaine O'Brien	Evergreen, Colorado
Julee O'Neil	Seattle, Washington
Bruce Pace	College Station, Texas
Paulette Financial Arrangements & Assoc.	Seattle, Washington
Sheryl Payne	Issaquah, Washington

Gary N. Peterson   Carmel Valley, California
Philip H. & Anne S. Peterson   Seattle, Washington
Emily C. Pierce   Sacramento, California
Kathiren & Roy Poulos   San Francisco, California
Charles Rafi   Auckland, New Zealand
R. R. Raniga & Family   Durban, South Africa
John & Hollis Ryan   Mercer Island, Washington
Paul Schmidt   Mount Shasta, California
Martin Shaw   London, England
Dr. & Mrs. Norman Sober
      & Lon Sober   Baltimore, Maryland
Don & Clarice Tarasoff & Family   Sidney, B.C. Canada
Stewart A. Trimble   Calistoga, California
Carole Tyburski   El Segundo, California
Ann Waite   Santa Rosa, California
Van & Glendal Warren   Houston, Texas
Marcia T. Weed   Laguna Beach, California
Dr. & Mrs. Leonard Weisenthal   Boling Brook, Illinois
Mr. & Mrs. L. Westheimer   Teaneck, New Jersey
Larry E. Williams   San Francisco, California
Jolyon Wilson   Capetown, South Africa

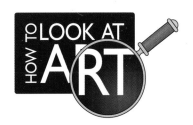

HOW TO LOOK AT ART

Showing Motion *in art*

Joy Richardson

Gareth Stevens Publishing
MILWAUKEE

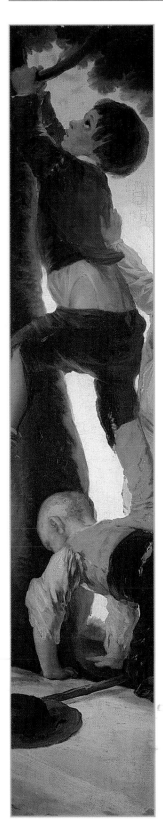

For a free color catalog describing Gareth Stevens' list of high-quality books and multimedia programs, call 1-800-542-2595 (USA) or 1-800-461-9120 (Canada). Gareth Stevens Publishing's Fax: (414) 225-0377.

Gareth Stevens Publishing would like to thank Gundega Spons of the Milwaukee Art Museum for her kind and professional help with the information in this book.

Library of Congress Cataloging-in-Publication Data available upon request from publisher.
Fax (414) 225-0377 for the attention of the Publishing Records Department.

ISBN 0-8368-2626-4

This North American edition first published in 2000 by
Gareth Stevens Publishing
1555 North RiverCenter Drive, Suite 201
Milwaukee, Wisconsin 53212 USA

Original edition © 1998 by Franklin Watts. First published in 1998 as *On the Move* by Franklin Watts, 96 Leonard Street, London, EC2A 4RH, United Kingdom. This U.S. edition © 2000 by Gareth Stevens, Inc. Additional end matter © 2000 by Gareth Stevens, Inc.

Gareth Stevens Editor: Monica Rausch
Gareth Stevens Cover Designer: Joel Bucaro
U.K. Editor: Sarah Ridley
U.K. Art Director: Robert Walster
U.K. Designer: White Design

Photographs: © The Ashmolean Museum, Oxford pp. 4-5, 26 (top); © by Courtesy of the Trustees of the British Museum pp. 16-17; © The Courtauld Institute pp. 22-23; © Kunsthistorisches Museum, Vienna cover, pp. 8-9, 27; reproduced by courtesy of the Trustees of the National Gallery, London pp. 10-11, 18-19, 20-21, 28, 30, 31; © Prado Museum pp. 14-15; Rochdale City Art Gallery/Bridgeman Art Library — 'Our Town' reproduced by courtesy of Mrs. Carol Ann Danes pp. 24-25; V&A Picture Library pp. 6-7, 26 (bottom); reproduced by permission of the Trustees of the Wallace Collection pp. 12-13.

Printed in Mexico

1 2 3 4 5 6 7 8 9 04 03 02 01 00

Contents

For additional information about the artists and paintings, see pages 30-31.

The Hunt in the Forest (*detail*)
painted by Paolo Uccello

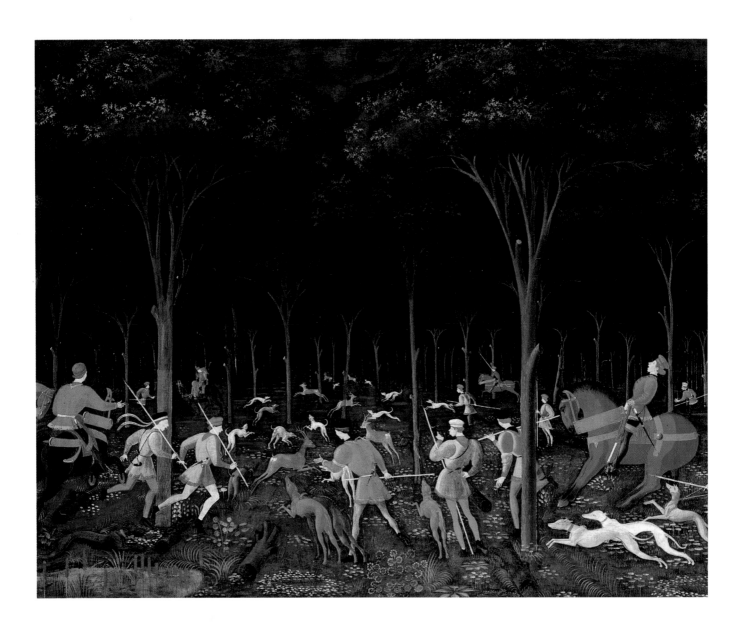

People, horses, and dogs jump and run. They are chasing deer into the deep, dark forest.

Dogs leap forward, stretching their bodies.

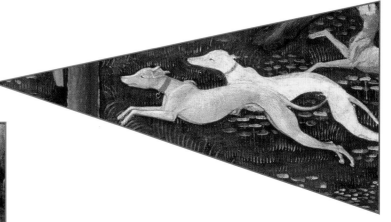

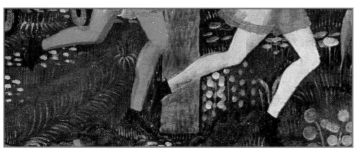

Legs bend and arms swing to help people run.

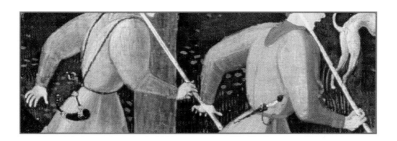

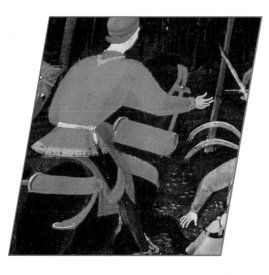

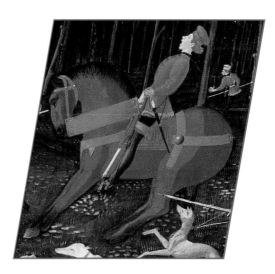

Who is moving forward, and who is stopping?

Night Attack on a Town
painted by Nafar Zamar

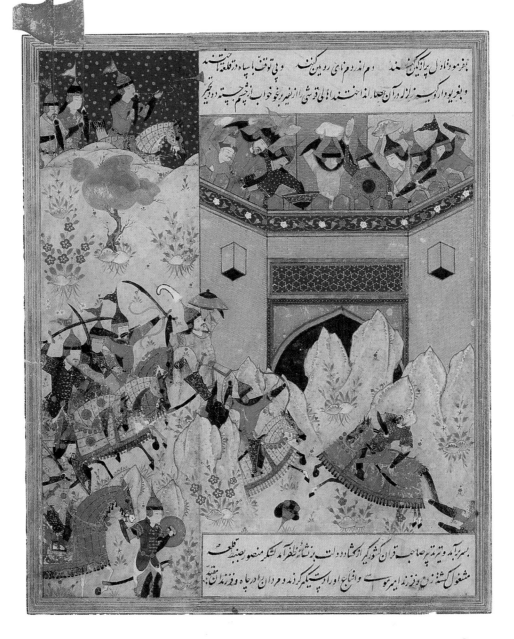

Enemy soldiers ride up to the gates of a town.
People fight to keep them out.

Horses prance in front of the gate.

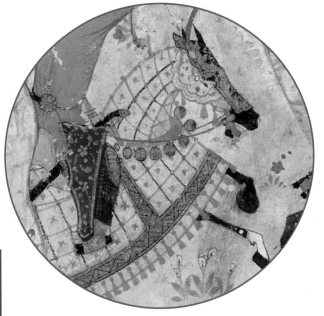

Archers aim their bows.

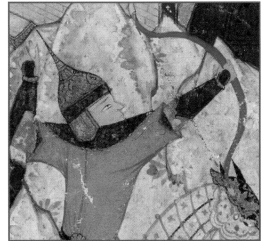

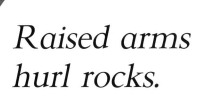

Raised arms hurl rocks.

Will this shield protect him?

Children's Games
painted by Pieter Bruegel

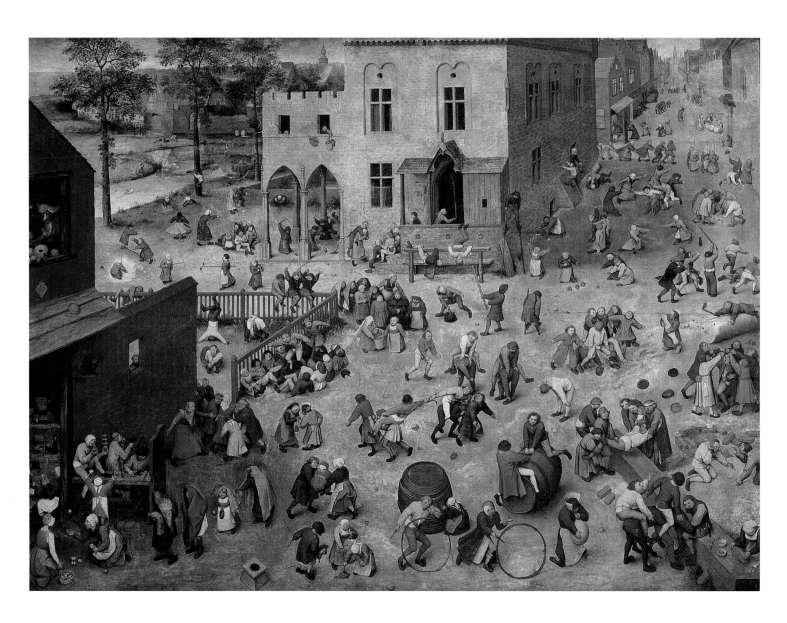

Two hundred children are busy playing.
Legs, arms, heads, and bodies all join in the games.

Look for children . . .

upside
down,

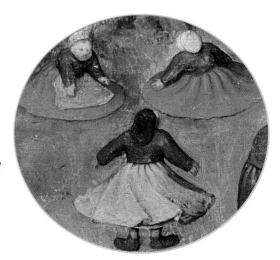

twirling
around,

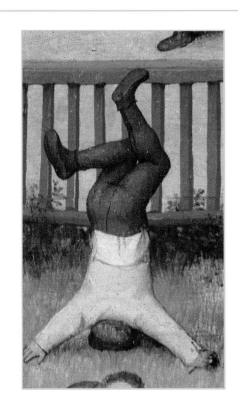

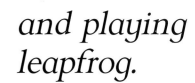

and playing
leapfrog.

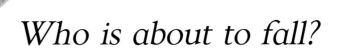

Who is about to fall?

A Winter Scene with Skaters
painted by Hendrick Avercamp

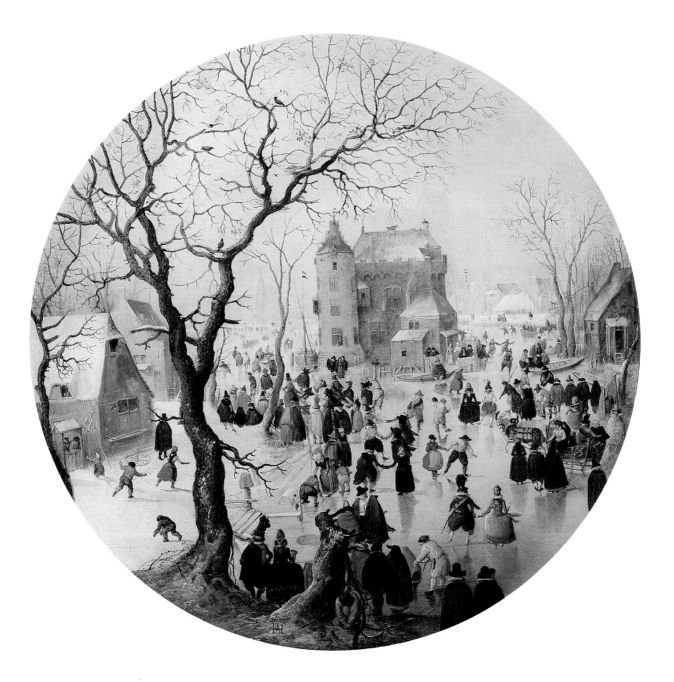

Everyone is out ice-skating and having fun.

Look for people . . .

kneeling
down,

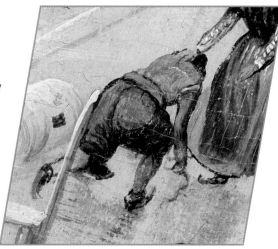

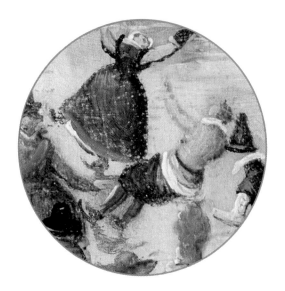

toppling
over,

skating along,

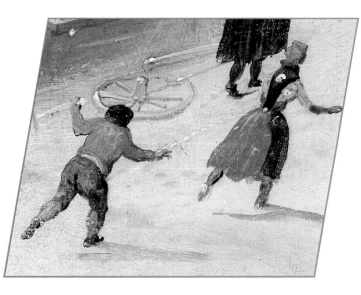

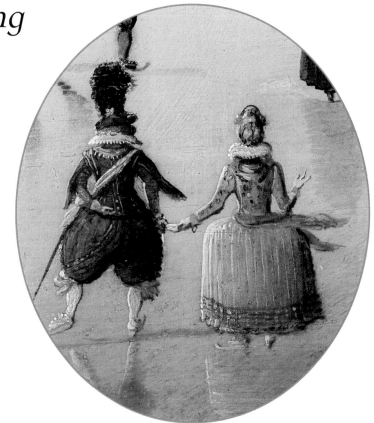

and dancing
on the ice.

The Swing
painted by Jean-Honoré Fragonard

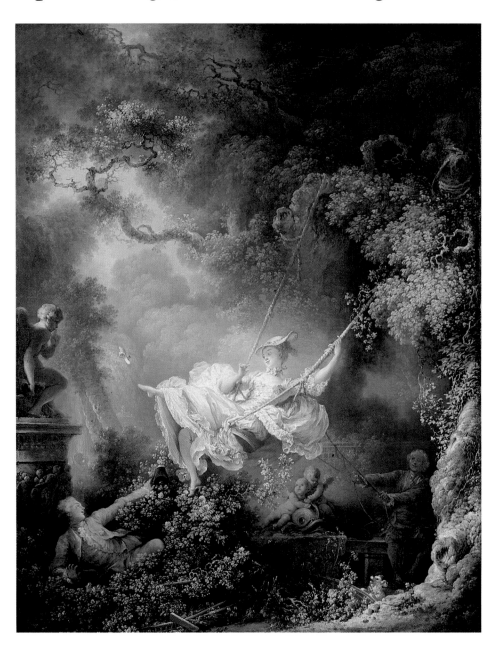

A beautiful young lady swings back
and forth under the trees.

Her pink dress
billows in the air.

She holds on
to the rope.

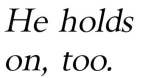

He holds
on, too.

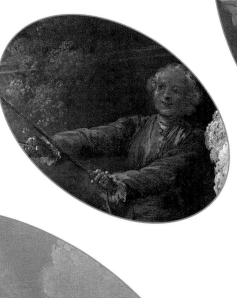

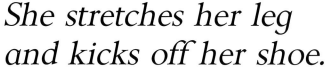

She stretches her leg
and kicks off her shoe.

Will her friend catch it?

Boys Climbing a Tree
painted by Francisco de Goya

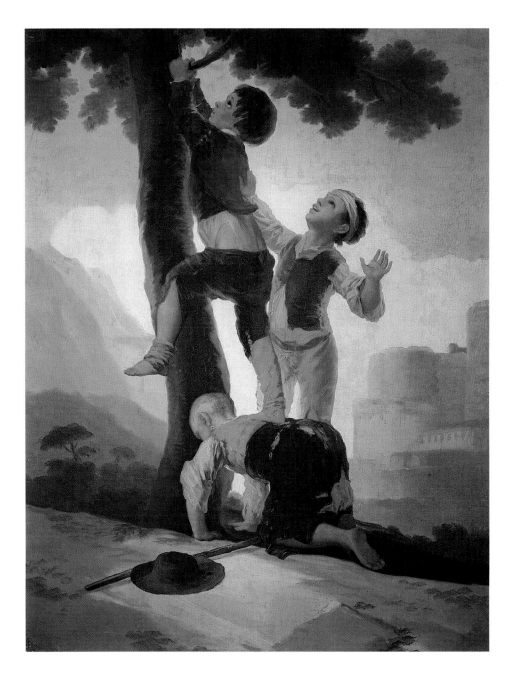

Two boys are helping their friend climb a tree.

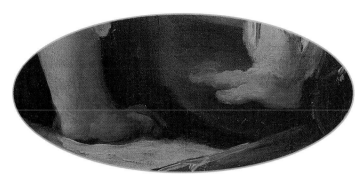

Hands press down
to hold the weight.

You can see
the back of a
small foot.

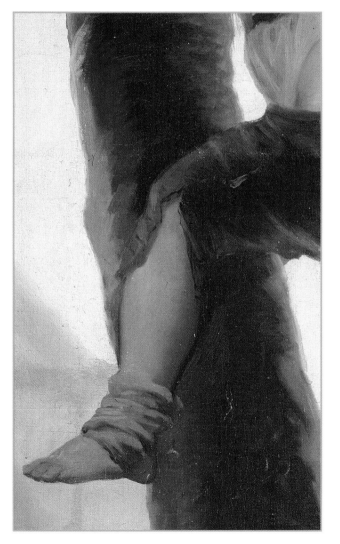

One leg
grips the
tree trunk.

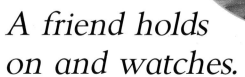

A friend holds
on and watches.

The Great Wave off Kanagawa
color print by Katsushika Hokusai

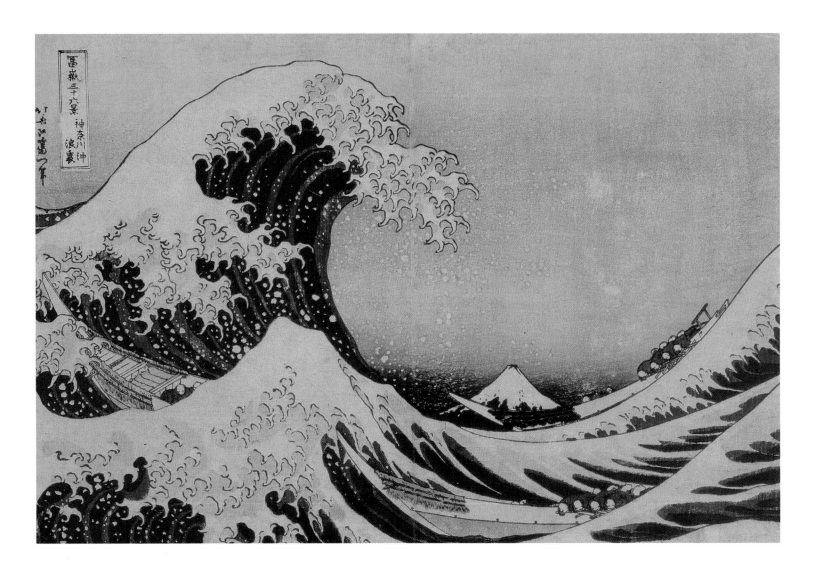

Surging, foaming waves curl and crash,
as boats cut through the water.

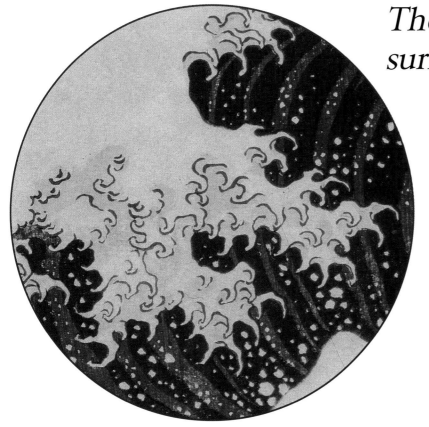

The wave rears up with surf like dragon claws.

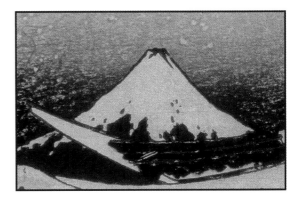

The waves frame a snow-capped mountain.

How many people can you see in the boats?

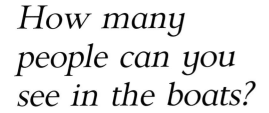

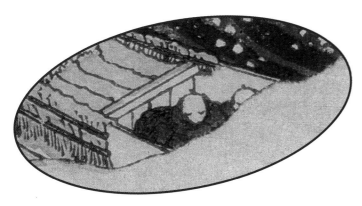

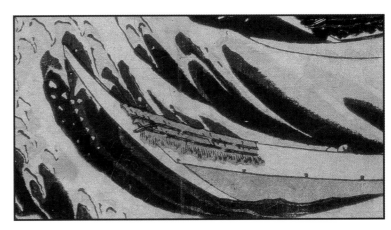

Where is the end of this boat?

La La at the Cirque Fernando
painted by Edgar Degas

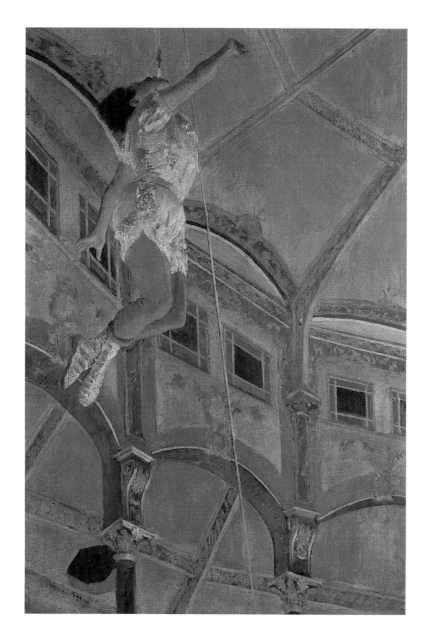

Degas loved painting people in action.
This acrobat is hanging high in the circus dome.

Can you see her holding
on by her teeth?

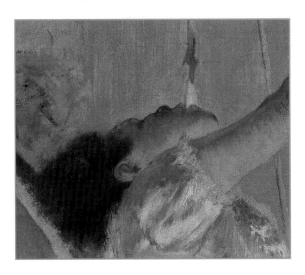

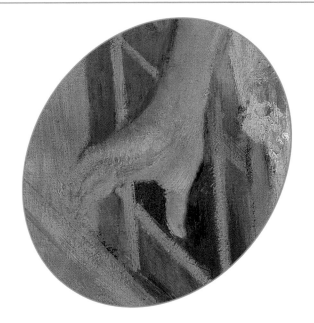

She balances with her
arms flung out.

Look at how she
bends her knees,

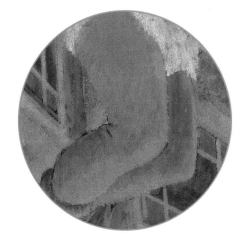

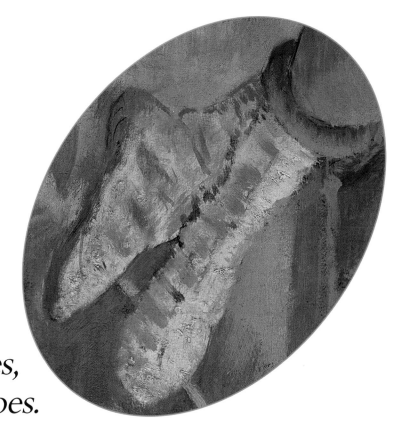

crosses her ankles,
and points her toes.

Tiger in a Tropical Storm (Surprise!)
painted by Henri Rousseau

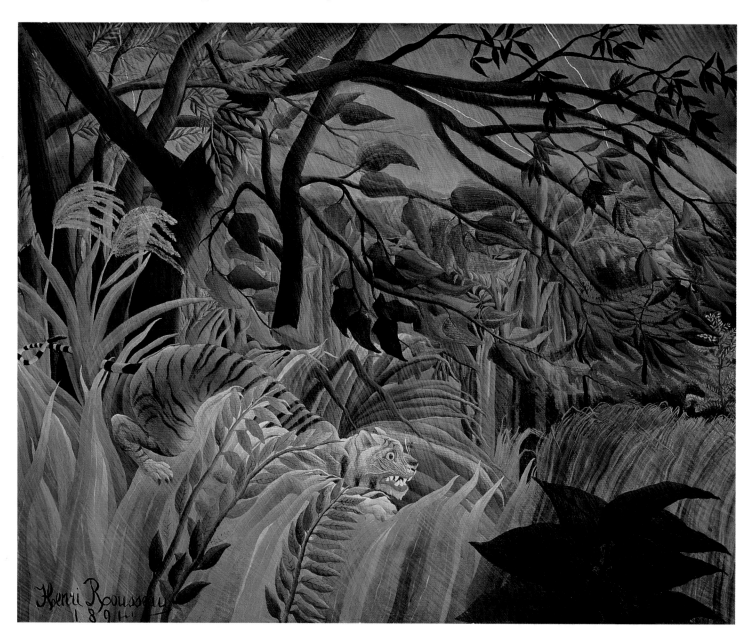

The tiger moves through the
forest as the rain lashes down.

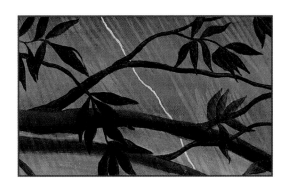

Can you see rain and lightning?

Follow the leaves to see which way the wind is blowing.

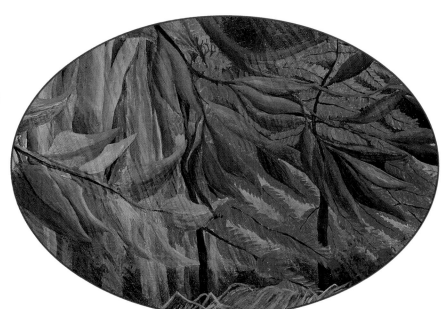

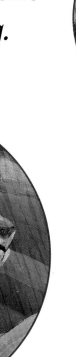

The tiger bounds through the undergrowth.

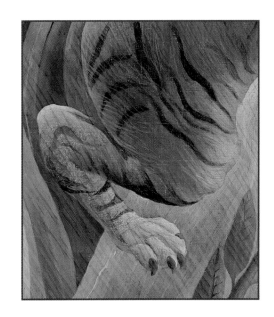

Look at its legs.

Study for Le Chahut
painted by Georges Seurat

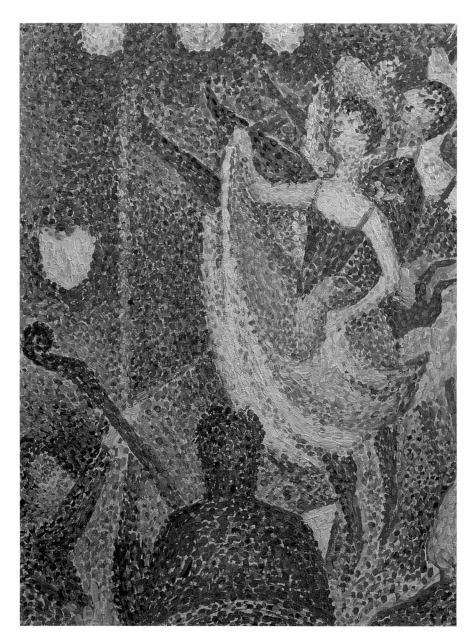

Dancers kick their legs as the music plays.
Seurat turns the scene into dots of color.

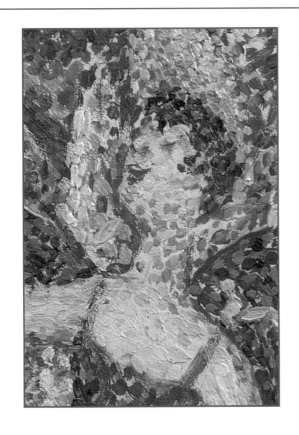

Her head leans back
as she kicks up high.

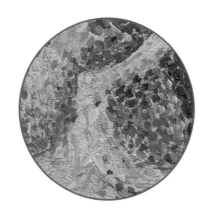

Look at the
hands holding
swirling skirts.

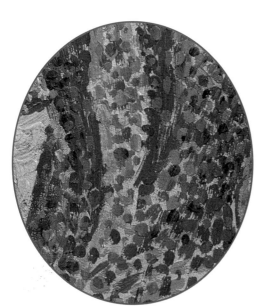

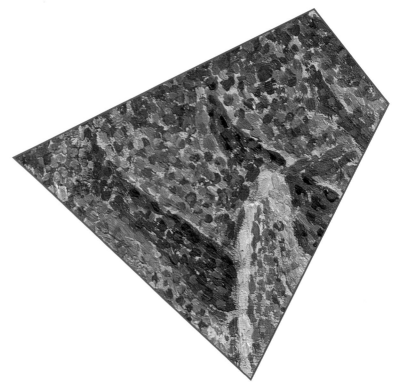

Can you match each
leg on the ground . . .

with a leg in the air?

Our Town
painted by L. S. Lowry

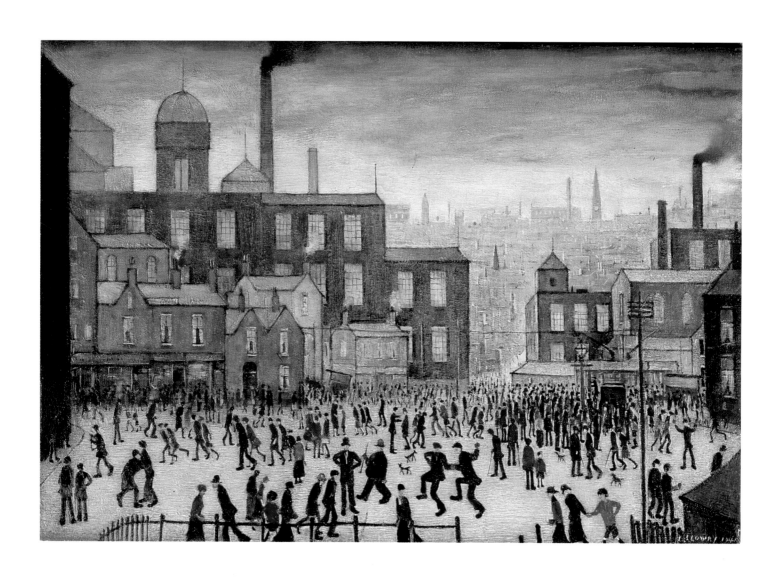

People hurry along or stand and
watch as the world goes by.

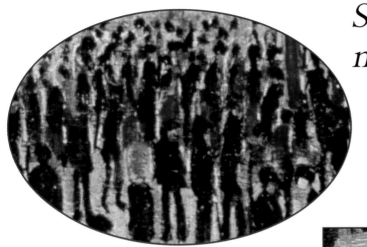

Strokes and dabs of brown make a crowd of people.

People walk briskly, leaning forward.

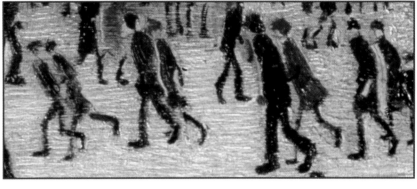

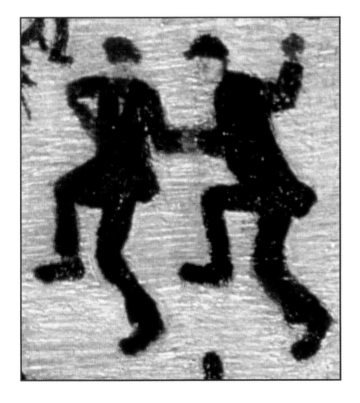

Arms and legs stand out against the pale background.

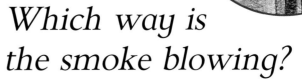

Which way is the smoke blowing?

Moving Parts

Knees bend

Look how legs bend when people run.

Try painting a group of runners to show what happens to their bodies when they run.

For help, look back at pages 4, 10, and 24.

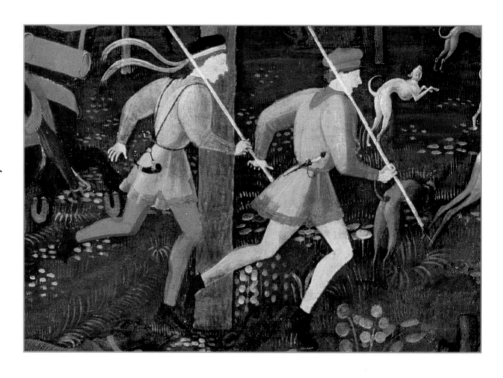

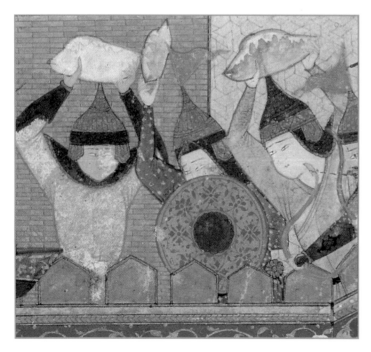

Arms stretch

How do arms move when people are running, throwing, reaching out, or holding on?

Try painting one of these actions with the arms in the right place.

For help, look back at pages 6, 8, 12, and 14.

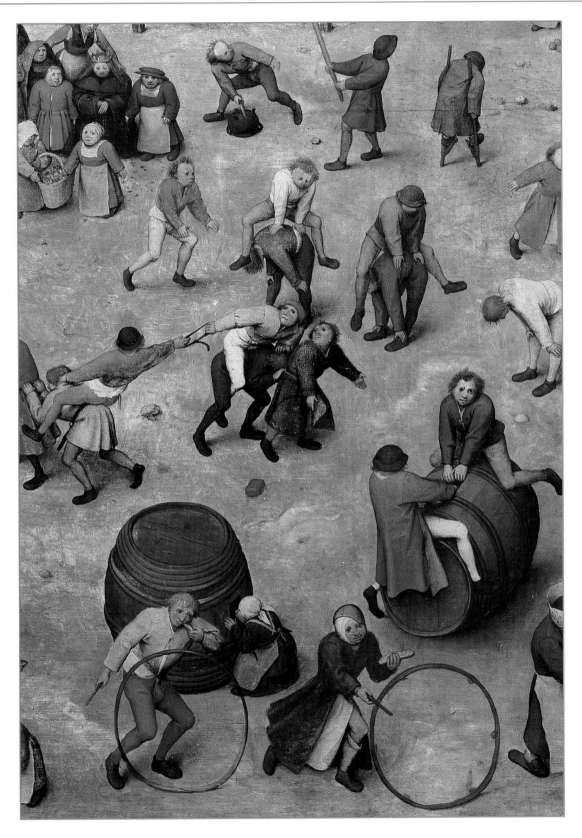

Bending bodies

Bodies in motion lean forward or backward, or twist or bend.

Paint a playground full of people, showing the shapes their bodies make as they play.

For help, look back at pages 8, 10, and 14.

Two legs or four?

How do animals move their legs?

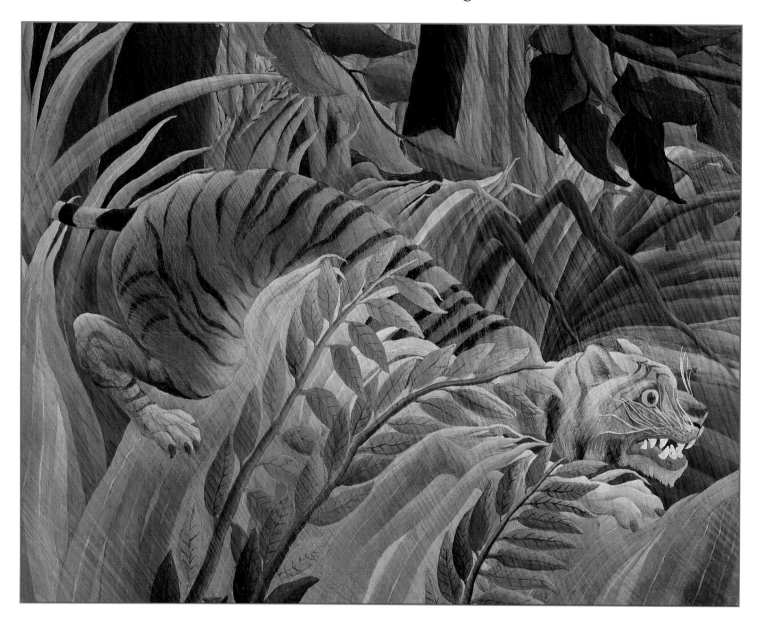

Try painting a cat, a horse, or a dog in motion.

For help, look back
at pages 4 and 20.

Seeing a pattern

Moving bodies make interesting shapes.

Make a simple drawing of someone running, dancing, or playing a game.

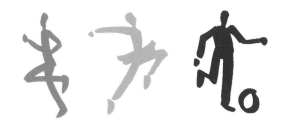

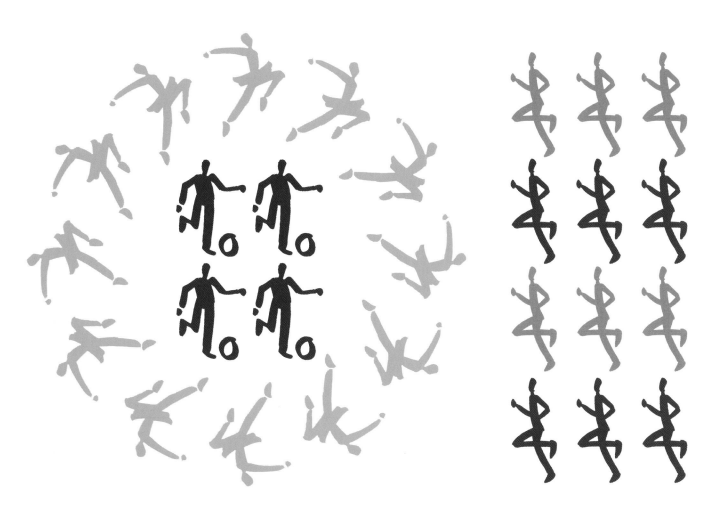

Repeat it to make an interesting pattern.
For help, look back at pages 8, 10, 22, and 24.

More about the paintings in this book

■ The Hunt in the Forest *(page 4)*

Paolo Uccello (1397-1475) lived in Florence. In this painting, he patterns the darkness with bright, moving figures. He was fascinated by the use of perspective and arranged the whole scene to draw the eye into the forest in pursuit of the deer.

■ Night Attack on a Town *(page 6)*

This picture is an illustration from *The Book of Victory* by Nafar Zamar, which celebrates the conquests of a Mogul Emperor. The Mogul Empire expanded in the sixteenth and seventeenth centuries to control much of India.

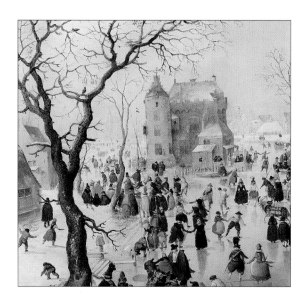

■ Children's Games *(page 8)*

Pieter Bruegel (about 1525-1569) the Elder lived in Holland. He had two sons, Jan and Pieter the Younger, who also became famous painters. He enjoyed painting the ordinary activities of village life, and he looked back with humor to the fun and games of his own childhood.

■ A Winter Scene with Skaters *(page 10)*

Hendrick Avercamp (1585-1634) lived in Holland, where low, flat land often flooded and froze in winter. Avercamp liked painting everyone coming out to enjoy themselves on the ice. Avercamp was deaf and could not speak, which perhaps made him observe life more sharply.

■ The Swing *(page 12)*

Jean-Honoré Fragonard (1732-1806) was a popular painter in Paris before the French Revolution. People liked his playful pictures of leisure and luxury. Here, a rich and fashionable young lady is teasing a suitor by kicking off her shoe for him to catch.

■ Boys Climbing a Tree *(page 14)*

Francisco de Goya (1746-1828) was Spanish. Goya often painted children, dressed in their best for formal portraits or simply playing naturally. This picture was one of a series painted on cardboard as designs for tapestries that were to be made at the royal factory.

■ The Great Wave off Kanagawa (page 16)

Katsushika Hokusai (1760-1849) was a Japanese artist. He responded to nature with simple but striking designs and colors. This color print is one of his *Thirty-six Views of Mount Fuji*. It shows Mount Fuji, an old volcano and the highest peak in Japan, through the hollow of a huge wave.

■ La La at the Cirque Fernando (page 18)

Edgar Degas (1834-1917) lived in Paris and loved painting entertainers at work. This painting shows an unusual view of La La, a circus acrobat who was famous for her strength, hanging from a wire by her teeth.

■ Tiger in a Tropical Storm (Surprise!) (page 20)

Henri Rousseau (1844-1910) learned all he could about exotic plants and animals without ever leaving France. He created this fantasy forest from his imagination, making a rich pattern of shapes and colors. He borrowed the tiger from a painting by another artist.

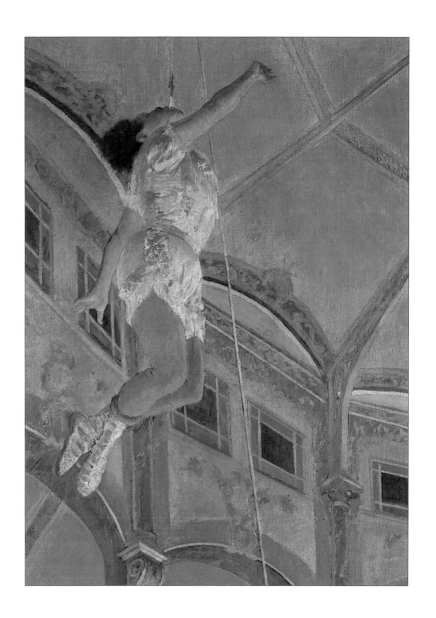

■ Study for Le Chahut (page 22)

Georges Seurat (1859-1891) was a French painter. He was interested in how our eyes see color and experimented with using separate dots or strokes of color to create an overall impression. He made this picture of high-kicking cabaret dancers in preparation for another painting.

■ Our Town (page 24)

L. S. Lowry (1887-1976) lived in northern England. He found beauty in city streets and crowds, factory buildings and smoking chimneys. He looked on as nameless people hurried about their business and painted them as dark figures against a light background.

Glossary

billows: rises in waves; swells out with air.

bustling: moving around busily or in an excited way.

hurl: throw.

impression: a feeling, memory, or image that sticks in the mind.

motion: movement; not staying still.

pattern: a decorative, usually repetitive, design.

perspective: showing objects on a flat surface as they appear spatially in real life.

portrait: a picture of a person's head or sometimes the person's entire body.

prance: to spring forward from the hind legs, stepping lively.

surging: rising and falling in waves; moving forward with a sudden force.

tapestries: a thick, heavy cloth woven with designs and scenes and hung on walls or over furniture.

toppling: falling over because of being too heavy on top.

Web Sites

Metropolitan Museum of Art Kids Page
www.metmuseum.org/htmlfile/education/kid.html

An Art Contest for Kids
www.artcontest.com/index.html

Due to the dynamic nature of the Internet, some web sites stay current longer than others. To find additional web sites, use a reliable search engine with one or more of the following keywords: *art, Edgar Degas, drawing animals, Katsushika Hokusai,* and *painting.*

Index